海峡两岸医药卫生交流协会银屑病专业委员会

Psoriasis Professional Committee of the Cross-Straits Medical and Health Exchange Association

成人寻常型银屑病医患共决策
——海峡两岸及港澳地区专家共识

Shared Decision-making between Physician and Patient in Adult Psoriasis Vulgaris

A Consensus among Experts Cross the Straits, Hong Kong and Macao

主　编　张晓艳

Editor-in-chief　Zhang Xiaoyan

副主编　钟文宏　张春雷　刘晓明

Subeditor　Chung Wenhung　Zhang Chunlei　Liu Xiaoming

U0224175

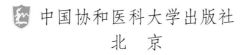

中国协和医科大学出版社

北　京

图书在版编目（CIP）数据

成人寻常型银屑病医患共决策：海峡两岸及港澳地区专家共识 / 张晓
艳主编 . —北京：中国协和医科大学出版社，2024.3（2025.4重印）.
ISBN 978-7-5679-2365-2

Ⅰ.①成⋯　Ⅱ.①张⋯　Ⅲ.①银屑病—诊疗　Ⅳ.①R758.63

中国国家版本馆 CIP 数据核字（2024）第 053380 号

主　　编　张晓艳
责任编辑　杨小杰　栾　韬
封面设计　邱晓俐
责任校对　张　麓
责任印制　黄艳霞
出版发行　**中国协和医科大学出版社**
　　　　　（北京市东城区东单三条 9 号　邮编 100730　电话 010-65260431）
网　　址　www.pumcp.com
印　　刷　鸿博睿特（天津）印刷科技有限公司
开　　本　889mm×1194mm　1/32
印　　张　4
字　　数　120 千字
版　　次　2024 年 3 月第 1 版
印　　次　2025 年 4 月第 2 次印刷
定　　价　52.00 元

编者名单

主　编　张晓艳

副主编　钟文宏　张春雷　刘晓明

编　者（按姓氏汉语拼音排序）

陈朝霞（首都医科大学附属北京中医医院　北京市中医药研究所）

陈俊宾（台湾林口长庚纪念医院）

范嘉仪（澳门仁伯爵综合医院）

侯素春（深圳大学总医院）

黄思敏（香港大学玛丽医院）

黄毓惠（台湾林口长庚纪念医院）

蓝政哲（台湾高雄医学大学附设中和纪念医院）

李　萍（首都医科大学附属北京中医医院　北京市中医药研究所）

刘晓明（华中科技大学协和深圳医院）

柳曦光（黑龙江省医院）

陆乃明（香港皮肤医学慈善基金会）

苗朝阳（国家儿童医学中心　首都医科大学附属北京儿童医院）

庞晓文（中国人民解放军空军特色医学中心）

夏建新（吉林大学第二医院）

张　睿（黑龙江省医院）

张春雷（北京大学第三医院）

张思亮（澳门仁伯爵综合医院）

张晓艳（中日友好医院）

钟文宏（台湾林口长庚纪念医院）

禚风麟（首都医科大学附属北京友谊医院）

绘　图　王丽华

Editor´s List

Wen-Hung Chung (Chang Gung Memorial Hospital, Linkou, Taiwan)

Xia Jianxin (The second hospital of Jilin University)

Yu-Huei Huang (Chang Gung Memorial Hospital, Linkou, Taiwan)

Zhang Chunlei (Peking University Third Hospital)

Zhang Rui (Heilongjiang province hospital)

Zhang Xiaoyan (China-Japan Friendship Hospital)

Zhuo Fenglin (Beijing Friendship Hospital, Capital Medical University)

Graphic editor   Wang Lihua

编者简介

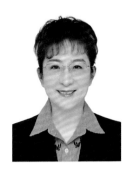

张晓艳

教授，博士研究生导师。

中日友好医院皮肤科主任医师/皮肤健康研究所副所长，海峡两岸医药卫生交流协会常务理事，海峡两岸医药卫生交流协会银屑病专业委员会主任委员，中国老年医学学会理事，中国女医师协会皮肤病分会常委等。

擅长银屑病与皮肤肿瘤防治和皮肤美容治疗等。主持银屑病相关国家自然科学基金等9项，发表论文90余篇，SCI收录19篇，获学术奖励多项，荣获"中国好医生""人民好医生"等国家/省部级奖多项，培养硕士及博士研究生35名。

Zhang Xiaoyan

Professor, PhD supervisor.

Chief physician of the Department of Dermatology at the China-Japan Friendship Hospital/Vice Director of the Institute of Skin Health, Standing Committee Member of the Cross-Strait Medical and Health Exchange Association, Chair of the Psoriasis Professional Committee of the Cross-Strait Medical and Health Exchange Association, Member of the Chinese Geriatrics Society, Standing Committee Member of the Dermatology Branch of the Chinese Medical Women's Association, etc.

Specializes in the prevention and treatment of psoriasis, skin tumors, and dermatological cosmetic treatments. Has led nine projects including the National Natural Science Foundation of China related to psoriasis, published over 90 papers, including 19 SCI papers, and has received numerous academic awards. Honored with multiple national/provincial level awards such as "China's Good Doctor" and "People's Good Doctor", and has supervised the training of 35 doctoral and master's students.

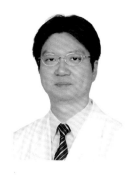

钟文宏

　　教授，台湾林口长庚纪念医院皮肤部部长，长庚医院药物过敏中心主任，台湾长庚医院基因体医学中心主任，台湾长庚大学医学系教授，厦门长庚医院副院长。法国皮肤科医学会荣誉会员。李镇源教授医学研究青年学者奖，第一届永信李天德医药科技杰出论文奖，2006年台湾十大潜力人物，长庚医院董事长金牌奖章，吴大猷先生纪念奖，台湾第47届十大杰出青年，台湾"科技部"2014年度杰出研究奖，国际皮肤科医学会联盟（ILDS）年轻医师成就奖等。

Zhong Wenhong

　　Professor. Chief of the Department of Dermatology at Chang Gung Memorial Hospital in Taiwan, Director of the Drug Hypersensitivity Center at Chang Gung Hospital, Director of the Genomic Medicine Center at Chang Gung Hospital, Professor in the Department of Medicine at Chang Gung University in Taiwan, Vice President of Xiamen Chang Gung Hospital. Honorary Member of the French Society of Dermatology. Recipient of the Li Chen-Yuan Professor Medical Research Young Scholar Award, the 1st Yongxin Li Tiande Outstanding Paper Award in Medical Science and Technology, named one of the Top Ten Potential Persons in Taiwan in 2006, awarded the President's Gold Medal from Chang Gung Hospital, recipient of the Wu Ta-You Memorial Award, named one of the Top Ten Outstanding Young People in the 47th Taiwan Ten Outstanding Young Persons, recipient of the Outstanding Research Award in 2014, and recipient of the Young Physician Achievement Award from the International League of Dermatological Societies (ILDS), among others.

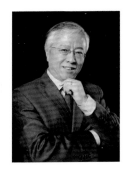

张春雷

　　北京医科大学医学博士，瑞士苏黎世大学医院和美国得州大学MD安德森癌症中心博士后。现任北京大学第三医院皮肤科主任医师、特聘教授（国家二级）和博士生导师。曾任北京大学第三医院皮肤科主任、北京大学皮肤科学系主任和美国MD安德森癌症中心皮肤科助理教授。现为亚洲银屑病学会理事、中华医学会皮肤性病学分会银屑病学组副组长和海峡两岸医药卫生交流协会银屑病专业委员会副主任委员。擅长皮肤肿瘤和免疫炎症性皮肤病的诊断治疗。

Zhang Chunlei

　　M.D., Ph.D. from Peking University Health Science Center, completed postdoctoral training at University Hospital Zurich in Switzerland and MD Anderson Cancer Center in the United States. Currently serves as Chief Physician, Tenured Professor (National Level), and Ph.D. Supervisor in the Department of Dermatology at Peking University Third Hospital. Formerly served as Director of the Dermatology Department at Peking University Third Hospital, Chair of the Department of Dermatology at Peking University, and Assistant Professor in Dermatology at MD Anderson Cancer Center in the United States. Currently holds positions as Director of the Asian Psoriasis Association, Deputy Leader of the Psoriasis Group of the Dermatology Branch of the Chinese Medical Association, and Vice Chairman of the Psoriasis Professional Committee of the Cross-Strait Medical and Health Exchange Association. Specializes in the diagnosis and treatment of skin tumors and immune-inflammatory skin diseases.

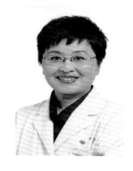

刘晓明

博士，博士生导师，国家二级教授，享受国务院特殊津贴专家。华中科技大学协和深圳医院皮肤科教授。曾任香港大学深圳医院科教总监，皮肤科负责人；中华医学会皮肤科分会12～14届常委；亚洲银屑病学会（ASP）理事；海峡两岸医疗促进会银屑病专委会副主委；*Dermatolodica Threapy* 学术编辑。从事皮肤科临床教学科研40余年，获省科技进步二等奖2项，三等奖3项；主持国家自然科学基金课题3项，省部级课题8项；发表学术论文160余篇。

Liu Xiaoming

Ph.D., doctoral supervisor, National Level Professor; enjoys special government allowances from the State Council. Professor of Dermatology at Huazhong University of Science and Technology Union Shenzhen Hospital. Formerly served as the Director of Science and Education and Head of the Dermatology Department at the University of Hong Kong Shenzhen Hospital; Member of the Dermatology Branch of the Chinese Medical Association for the 12th to 14th sessions; Director of the Asian Psoriasis Association (ASP); Vice Chairman of the Psoriasis Professional Committee of the Cross-Strait Medical Promotion Association; Academic Editor of "*Dermatological Therapy*". Engaged in clinical teaching and research in dermatology for over 40 years, won two second prizes and three third prizes for provincial scientific and technological progress; led three projects funded by the National Natural Science Foundation and eight projects at the provincial and ministerial levels; published over 160 academic papers.

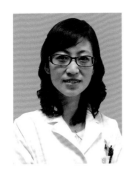

陈朝霞

副研究员，副教授，硕士研究生导师。首都医科大学附属北京中医医院北京市中医药研究所，第六批北京市级中医药专家学术经验继承人。任中国民族医药学会皮肤病分会理事、北京中医药学会外治专业委员会委员。从事中医治疗皮肤科疾病医教研10余年，擅长银屑病、特应性皮炎、白癜风等的诊治与研究。获中华中医药学会科学技术三等奖2项，主持及参与课题10余项，发表中英文论文20余篇，授权专利9项，参编专著12部。

Chen Zhaoxia

Associate Researcher, Associate Professor, Master's Supervisor. Affiliated with Beijing Hospital of Traditional Chinese Medicine, Beijing Institute of Traditional Chinese Medicine, Capital Medical University. Designated as one of the sixth batch of Beijing municipal−level experts in traditional Chinese medicine. Serves as a Director of the Dermatology Branch of the Chinese Society of Ethnic Medicine and Beijing Society of Traditional Chinese Medicine's External Treatment Professional Committee. Engaged in teaching, clinical practice, and research in traditional Chinese medicine dermatology for over 10 years, specializing in the diagnosis and treatment of psoriasis, atopic dermatitis, vitiligo, etc. Received two third prizes from the China Association of Chinese Medicine for Science and Technology, led and participated in over 10 research projects, published over 20 papers in both Chinese and English, holds 9 authorized patents, and contributed to the compilation of 12 monographs.

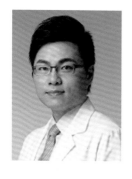

陈俊宾

助理教授级主治医师。任职于台湾林口长庚医院皮肤部及医学美容中心，药物过敏临床与研究中心主任，在长庚大学和清华大学授课。海峡两岸医药卫生交流协会银屑病专委会常委兼副秘书长，台湾医用激光光电学会会员，台湾皮肤科医学会美容专科训练认证医师，台湾皮肤科医学会皮肤镜训练认证，台湾皮肤科医学会会员。台湾皮肤医学会和台湾皮肤研究医学会官方期刊 *Dermatologica Sinica* 执行副编辑，获2022年台湾吴大猷先生纪念奖，2022年日本皮肤病研究学会青年学者奖。发表学术论文100余篇。

Chen Junbin   Assistant Professor-level Attending Physician. Works at the Department of Dermatology and Medical Cosmetology Center of Chang Gung Hospital in Taiwan, serving as Director of the Clinical and Research Center for Drug Allergy and teaching at Chang Gung University and Tsinghua University. Also, he is a standing committee member and deputy secretary-general of the Psoriasis Committee of the Cross-Strait Medical and Health Exchange Association, a member of the Taiwan Medical Laser and Optoelectronics Association, a certified physician in cosmetic dermatology by the Taiwan Dermatological Association, certified in dermatoscopy by the Taiwan Dermatological Association, and a member of the Taiwan Dermatological Association. He serves as the Associate Editor of the official journals of the Taiwan Dermatological Society and the Taiwan Society for Investigative Dermatology, "*Dermatologica Sinica*". He received the Mr. Wu Ta-You Memorial Award of Taiwan in 2022 and the Young Scholar Award from the Japanese Society for Investigative Dermatology in 2022. He has published over 100 academic papers.

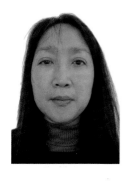

范嘉仪

澳门仁伯爵综合医院皮肤科首席顾问医生。2004年在该院完成皮肤科培训，成为皮肤科专科医生。澳门医学专科学院皮肤科院士，《澳门医学杂志》编辑，澳门医护志愿者协会会务顾问医生，澳门皮肤学会理事，香港皮肤性病学会员，葡萄牙皮肤性病学会员。

Fan Jiayi　Chief Consultant Dermatologist at Conde de São Januário Hospital Center in Macau. Completed dermatology training at the hospital in 2004 and became a specialist dermatologist. Fellow of the Macau Academy of Medical Specialties in Dermatology, Editor of *"the Macau Medical Journal"*, Executive Advisor Doctor of the Macau Medical and Nursing Volunteers Association, Director of the Macau Dermatological Society, member of the Hong Kong Society of Dermatology and Venereology, and member of the Portuguese Society of Dermatology and Venereology.

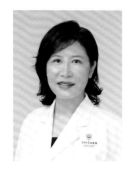

侯素春

医学博士，主任医师，硕士研究生导师。深圳大学总医院皮肤科主任。美国亨利福特医院访问学者，2016年7月赴香港大学玛丽医院及香港皮肤激光中心研修。从事临床工作30年，擅长银屑病、特应性皮炎、重症药疹等复杂重症皮肤病的诊断与治疗。主持和参与省级、国家级科研课题多项，在核心期刊及SCI收录期刊发表学术论文30余篇，获辽宁省科技进步二等奖一项。

Hou Suchun　Doctor of Medicine, Chief Physician, Master's Supervisor. Director of the Dermatology Department at Shenzhen University General Hospital. Visiting Scholar at Henry Ford Hospital in the United States, underwent training at Queen Mary Hospital and the Hong Kong Skin Laser Center of the University of Hong Kong in July 2016. Engaged in clinical work for 30 years, specializing in the diagnosis and treatment of complex and severe skin diseases such as psoriasis, atopic dermatitis, and severe drug eruptions. Has led and participated in several provincial and national research projects, published over 30 academic papers in core journals and SCI journals, and won one second prize for scientific and technological progress in Liaoning Province.

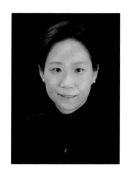

黄思敏

　　医学硕士，副教授，毕业于香港大学，玛丽医院皮肤科主任，香港大学名誉临床副教授。以优异的成绩获得伦敦国王学院圣约翰皮肤病研究所临床皮肤病学硕士学位，并获得香港医学专科学院和英国爱丁堡皇家医学院的院士资格。香港皮肤性病学会主席及香港皮肤科专科学院名誉秘书。主要研究包括特应性皮炎、银屑病和皮肤药疹的先进治疗。一直与中国（包括香港）的各个患者团体和协会密切合作，以促进医疗保健。

Huang Simin　Master of Medicine, Associate Professor. Graduated from the University of Hong Kong. Director of the Dermatology Department at Queen Mary Hospital and Honorary Clinical Associate Professor at the University of Hong Kong. Achieved outstanding results and obtained a Master's degree in Clinical Dermatology from the St John's Institute of Dermatology at King's College London. Holds fellowship qualifications from the Hong Kong Academy of Medicine and the Royal College of Physicians of Edinburgh. Serves as the Chairperson of the Hong Kong Society of Dermatology and the Honorary Secretary of the Hong Kong College of Dermatologists. Her primary research focuses on advanced treatments for atopic dermatitis, psoriasis, and drug eruptions. She has closely collaborated with various patient groups and associations in China（including Hong Kong）to promote healthcare.

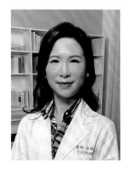

黄毓惠

副教授，医学博士，台北林口长庚纪念医院皮肤科副主任，副教授级主治医师，长庚大学副教授，长庚技术学院化妆品应用学系讲师，台湾皮肤科医学会理事及发言人，台湾干癣暨皮肤免疫学会常务理事，台湾卫福部食药署化妆品卫生管理资议会委员，台湾皮肤科医学会会员，台湾皮肤暨美容外科医学会会员，美国皮肤科医学会会员。

Huang Yuhui Associate Professor, Doctor of Medicine. Deputy Director and Associate Professor-level Attending Physician at the Department of Dermatology, Taipei Chang Gung Memorial Hospital, Linkou Branch. Also serves as an Associate Professor at Chang Gung University and Lecturer at the Department of Cosmetic Applications at Chang Gung Institute of Technology. Holds positions as a Director and spokesperson for the Taiwan Dermatological Association, Executive Director of the Taiwanese Psoriasis and Skin Immunology Society, Committee Member of the Cosmetics Hygiene Management Advisory Council under the Taiwan Food and Drug Administration of the Ministry of Health and Welfare, and is a member of the Taiwan Dermatological Association, the Taiwan Society of Dermatologic and Aesthetic Surgery, and the American Academy of Dermatology.

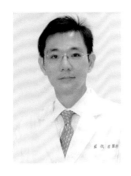

蓝政哲

　　教授。台湾高雄医学大学医学系皮肤科教授，高雄医学大学附设中和纪念医院皮肤部主任。台湾皮肤科医学会常务董事，色素细胞学会国际联合协会理事，亚洲色素细胞研究会院长。《光皮肤学》《光免疫学》和《光医学》主编，《皮肤科杂志》章节编辑。

Lan Zhengzhe　　Prof. Professor of Dermatology, Department of Medicine, Kaohsiung Medical University (KMU), Taiwan, and Director of the Department of Dermatology, Chung-Ho Memorial Hospital attached to KMU. Managing Director of the Taiwan Dermatology Medical Association, Director of the International Joint Association of Pigment Cell Societies, and President of the Asian Pigment Cell Research Society. Editor-in-Chief of *"Photodermatology" "Photo-Immunology"* and *"Photomedicine"* and Chapter Editor of *"Journal of Dermatology"*.

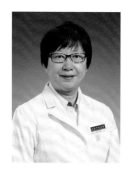

李萍

研究员，教授，博士生导师。北京市中医药研究所副所长。创建国家中医药管理局"疮疡生肌理论及应用"重点研究室、国家中医药管理局"细胞病理"三级实验室和"银屑病中医临床基础研究北京市重点实验室"。中国病理生理学会副理事长兼秘书长，北京中医药学会中医外科专业委员会副主任委员。主要开展中西医结合治疗银屑病、难愈性创面、特应性皮炎/湿疹、白癜风等难治性皮肤病的研究。承担国家级、省部级以上课题10余项，著作3部，成果8项，专利7项，论文160篇。

Li Ping researcher, professor, doctoral supervisor. Deputy Director of Beijing Institute of Traditional Chinese Medicine. She is the founder of the State Administration of Traditional Chinese Medicine (SATCM) Key Research Laboratory of "Theory and Application of Sores and Muscle Regeneration", the State Administration of Traditional Chinese Medicine (SATCM) Level III Laboratory of "Cellular Pathology", and the Beijing Key Laboratory of Clinical and Basic Research on Psoriasis in Chinese Medicine. " She is the vice director of the Chinese Society of Pathophysiology. She is the vice president and secretary general of the Chinese Society of Pathophysiology, and the vice chairman of the TCM Surgery Committee of the Beijing Society of Traditional Chinese Medicine. She mainly carries out research on the combination of Chinese and Western medicine in the treatment of psoriasis, difficult-to-heal wounds, atopic dermatitis/eczema, vitiligo and other difficult-to-treat skin diseases. She has undertaken more than 10 national, provincial and ministerial level projects, 3 books, 8 achievements, 7 patents and 160 papers.

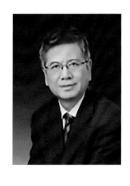

柳曦光

主任医师，研究生导师，哈工大兼职教授。黑龙江省医院皮肤病医院院长。1984年毕业于河北医科大学。省级领军人才梯队学科带头人，首届龙江名医。中华医学会皮肤病学分会全国委员、皮肤病理学组副组长，中国医师协会皮肤科医师分会常务委员，海峡两岸医药卫生交流协会银屑病专委会副主任委员，世界华人医师协会皮肤科医师协会常务委员，中国医疗保健国际交流促进会皮肤科分会常务委员。《实用皮肤病学》《临床皮肤科》《中华皮肤科杂志》编委；参与编写多部国家级教材。国内外杂志及学术会议发表论文60余篇。

Liu Xiguang   Chief Physician, Postgraduate Supervisor, Part-time Professor of HITS. Director of Dermatology Hospital of Heilongjiang Provincial Hospital. He graduated from Hebei Medical University in 1984. Provincial leading talent team discipline leader, the first Longjiang Famous Doctor. He is a national member of the Dermatology Branch of the Chinese Medical Association and deputy head of the Dermatopathology Group, an executive member of the Dermatologists Branch of the Chinese Physicians Association, a vice chairman of the Psoriasis Specialized Committee of the Cross-Strait Medicine and Health Exchange Association, an executive member of the Dermatologists Association of the World Association of Chinese Physicians, and an executive member of the Dermatology Branch of the China Association for the Promotion of International Exchanges in Healthcare. He is a member of the editorial boards of "*Practical Dermatology*" "*Clinical Dermatology*" and "*Chinese Journal of Dermatology*", and has participated in the preparation of several national textbooks. He has published more than 60 papers in domestic and international journals and academic conferences.

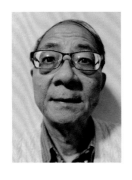

陆乃明

香港皮肤医学慈善基金会

医生，1987年毕业于香港中文大学医学系。他在英国圣约翰皮肤病研究所进一步深造，成绩卓越。自1998年起，他相继成为香港医学专科学院、香港内科医学院及英国皇家内科和外科医生学院的院士。在2004年至2013年期间，他担任香港中文大学皮肤科研究中心主任，并于2016年开始担任香港皮肤科基金会主席。此外，2006年他加入了香港皮肤性病学会理事会。

陆博士拥有超过25年的社会卫生科工作经验，他的研究兴趣广泛，包括皮肤癌、职业性皮肤病、痤疮和特应性皮炎等领域。他的研究成果已在《临床与实验皮肤病学》《接触性皮炎》和《欧洲皮肤病学与性病学会杂志》等国际知名期刊上发表。

Lu Naiming graduated from the Department of Medicine at the Chinese University of Hong Kong in 1987. He further pursued his studies at the St. John's Institute of Dermatology in the UK, achieving outstanding results. Since 1998, he has been a Fellow of the Hong Kong Academy of Medicine, the Hong Kong College of Physicians and the Royal College of Physicians and Surgeons of the United Kingdom. He was the Director of the Dermatology Research Center of the Chinese University of Hong Kong from 2004 to 2013 and has been the Chairman of the Hong Kong Dermatology Foundation since 2016. In addition, he joined the Council of the Hong Kong Society of Dermatology and Venereology in 2006.

Dr. Lu has over 25 years of experience working in the Social Hygiene Department. His research interests are wide-ranging and include the areas of skin cancer, occupational skin diseases, acne and atopic dermatitis. His research findings have been published in internationally recognized journals such as *"Clinical and Experimental Dermatology" "Contact Dermatitis"* and *"Journal of the European Society of Dermatology and Venereology"*.

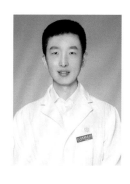

苗朝阳

医学博士，主治医师。就职于首都医科大学附属北京儿童医院皮肤科。从事儿童皮肤病的诊疗工作，主要研究方向为银屑病的临床和发病机制研究。主持国家自然科学基金青年项目1项，核心期刊及SCI收录期刊发表学术论文10余篇。

Chaoyang Miao is an attending physician. Dr. Miao works in the Department of Dermatology, Beijing Children's Hospital, Capital Medical University. Dr. Miao is engaged in the diagnosis and treatment of pediatric dermatology, and his main research interests are the clinical and pathogenesis of psoriasis. Hosted a youth project funded by the National Natural Science Foundation of China, and published over 10 academic papers in core journals and SCI journals.

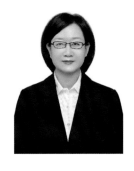

庞晓文

主任医师，教授，空军高层次科技人才，硕士研究生导师。中国人民解放军空军特色医学中心皮肤科，银屑病专科主任。1998年毕业于北京医科大学（现北京大学医学部）皮肤性病学专业，获医学博士学位。海峡两岸医药交流协会银屑病专业委员会副主任委员，北京医学会皮肤性病学分会委员，北京长江药学发展基金会理事。《中华皮肤科杂志》《解放军医学杂志》《人民军医》《空军医学》等审稿专家，北京市科委评审专家。发表SCI及国家期刊论文70余篇，副主编参编著作10部。

Pang Xiaowen　Chief Physician, Professor, High level Science and Technology Talent of the Air Force, Master's Supervisor. Director of the Department of Dermatology and Psoriasis Specialty at the Air Force Special Medical Center of the People's Liberation Army of China. Graduated from Beijing Medical University (now the Medical Department of Peking University) with a major in dermatology and venereology in 1998, and obtained a Doctor of Medicine degree. Vice Chairman of the Psoriasis Professional Committee of the Cross-Strait Medical and Health Exchange Association, Member of the Dermatology and Venereology Branch of the Beijing Medical Association, and Director of the Beijing Changjiang Pharmaceutical Development Foundation. She is a reviewer of "*Chinese Journal of Dermatology*" "*PLA Medical Journal*" "*People's Army Medicine*" "*Air Force Medicine*" etc. She is also a reviewer of Beijing Municipal Science and Technology Commission. She has published more than 70 papers in SCI and national journals, and has co-edited 10 books.

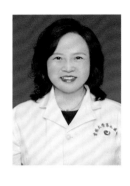

夏建新

　　教授、主任医师，医学博士，硕士研究生导师。吉林大学第二医院皮肤科副主任，日本九州大学皮肤科博士后。中华医学会病理学分会皮肤病理学组委员，中国中西医结合学会皮肤性病学分会银屑病学组委员，中国医师协会皮肤性病学分会皮肤病理学组委员，吉林省医师协会皮肤性病学分会副主任委员，海峡两岸医药卫生交流协会银屑病专委会常委。《中国皮肤性病学杂志》编委，吉林省医师协会皮肤性病学分会银屑病学组组长。擅长皮肤病理诊断以及银屑病的规范化治疗。

Xia Jianxin　Professor, Chief Physician, Doctor of Medicine, Master's Supervisor. Deputy Director of the Department of Dermatology, Second Hospital of Jilin University, and Postdoctoral Fellow in the Department of Dermatology, Kyushu University, Japan. Member of the Skin Pathology Group of the Pathology Branch of the Chinese Medical Association, Member of the Psoriasis Group of the Dermatology and Sexuality Branch of the Chinese Association of Traditional Chinese and Western Medicine, Member of the Skin Pathology Group of the Dermatology and Sexuality Branch of the Chinese Medical Association, Vice Chairman of the Dermatology and Sexuality Branch of the Jilin Medical Association, and Standing Committee Member of the Psoriasis Special Committee of the Cross Strait Medical and Health Exchange Association. Editorial board member of the *"Chinese Journal of Dermatology and Sexuality"*, and leader of the Psoriasis Group of the Dermatology and Sexuality Branch of the Jilin Medical Association. Proficient in skin pathological diagnosis and standardized treatment of psoriasis.

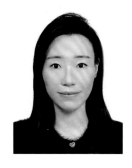

张思亮

主治医师，医学硕士。澳门仁伯爵综合医院皮肤科。2006年毕业于中山大学孙逸仙纪念医院，取得内科临床医学硕士学位。曾先后在澳门科技大学附属医院、澳门镜湖医院、澳门卫生局就职。并在澳门卫生局皮肤科专业基础培训实习、上海复旦大学华山医院皮肤科培训，并于2021年完成澳门仁伯爵综合医院皮肤科专科培训，工作至今。澳门医学专科学院皮肤科院士，《澳门医学杂志》编辑，澳门皮肤学会理事。

Zhang Siliang　attending physician, Master of Medicine. Department of Dermatology, Macao Hospital, Piaget Yan, graduated from Sun Yat-Sen Memorial Hospital of Sun Yat-Sen University in 2006 with a Master of Clinical Medicine degree in Internal Medicine. She has worked in Macao University of Science and Technology Hospital, Macao Kiang Wu Hospital and Macao Health Bureau. She also completed his basic training in dermatology at the Macau Health Bureau, her training in dermatology at Huashan Hospital of Fudan University in Shanghai, and completed her specialty training in dermatology at the Macau General Hospital in 2021, and has been working there since then. She is a Fellow of the Department of Dermatology of the Macao Academy of Medical Sciences, Editor of the *"Macao Medical Journal"* and Director of the Macao Dermatological Society.

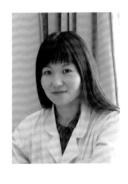

张睿

主任医师，硕士研究生导师。黑龙江省医院皮肤病医院银屑病诊疗中心主任。1997年毕业于中国医科大学，2004—2005年赴日本新潟研修。全球银屑病检测项目中国委员会委员，海峡两岸医药卫生交流协会银屑病专委会委员，中国中药协会皮肤病药物研究专业委员会银屑病、湿疹学组委员，黑龙江省慢病学会变态反应专委会副主任委员，黑龙江女医师协会常务理事、整形美容分会常务理事等。获省医药卫生科技进步三等奖，新技术二等奖、三等奖。

Zhang Rui　chief physician, master's supervisor. Director of the Psoriasis Diagnosis and Treatment Center at the Dermatology Hospital of Heilongjiang Province Hospital. Graduated from China Medical University in 1997 and went to Niigata, Japan for further studies from 2004 to 2005. Member of the Chinese Committee for Global Psoriasis Testing Project, member of the Psoriasis Special Committee of the Cross Strait Medical and Health Exchange Association, member of the Psoriasis and Eczema Group of the Dermatological Drug Research Professional Committee of the Chinese Association of Traditional Chinese Medicine, Vice Chairman of the Allergy Special Committee of the Heilongjiang Society of Chronic Diseases, Executive Director of the Heilongjiang Women's Physicians Association, and Executive Director of the Plastic Surgery and Cosmetic Branch. Received the third prize for provincial medical and health technology progress, as well as the second and third prizes for new technologies.

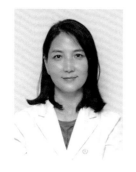

禚风麟

主任医师，教授，博士生导师。首都医科大学附属北京友谊医院皮肤科副主任。海峡两岸医药卫生交流协会银屑病专委会常委兼副秘书长，中华医学会皮肤性病学分会青年委员会委员、激光美容学组委员，中国整形美容协会形塑与综合技术转化分会副会长，中国抗衰老促进会医学美容专业委员会总干事等。主持国家自然基金2项、北京市自然基金3项、国家重点实验室基金等，专利3项，参编书籍4部，参写指南3篇，曾在悉尼大学、哈佛大学麻省总院访学。

Zhuo Fenglin　Chief Physician, Professor, Doctoral Supervisor. Deputy Director of the Dermatology Department of Beijing Friendship Hospital Affiliated to Capital Medical University. Member of the Standing Committee and Deputy Secretary General of the Psoriasis Special Committee of the Cross Strait Medical and Health Exchange Association, member of the Youth Committee and Laser Cosmetology Group of the Dermatology and Venereology Branch of the Chinese Medical Association, Vice President of the Shaping and Comprehensive Technology Transformation Branch of the China Plastic Surgery Association, and General Secretary of the Medical Cosmetology Professional Committee of the China Anti Aging Promotion Association. Presided over 2 projects of National Natural Science Foundation of China, 3 projects of Beijing Municipal Natural Science Foundation of China, State Key Laboratory Fund, etc; 3 patents; Participated in the compilation of four books; 3 guidebooks; Visited the University of Sydney and the Massachusetts Institute of Technology at Harvard University.

序

银屑病是一种慢性、复发性、炎症性、系统性疾病，以寻常型银屑病最为常见。除皮损外，银屑病患者罹患心血管疾病、代谢性疾病等系统共病的风险显著增加，给患者身心及其家庭和社会均带来沉重的负担。

近年来，随着银屑病发病机制研究的深入和生物医药技术的快速发展，生物制剂与小分子靶向药物相继问世，显著提高了患者的临床疗效，患者的结局和预后也得到明显改善。但是，疾病复发和共病进展并未得到有效遏制，伴随治疗而来的感染、过敏、继发性失应答等常常发生，患者对治疗方案的认知度不足，对治疗的依从性较低，使上述问题更加凸显。

如何根据患者的病情选择合理的个性化治疗方案、提高患者的依从性，使患者能够积极主动地接受科学规范的治疗，是防范和降低上述风险的关键，而医患双方有效对话、以医生为主导的医患双方共同决策，无疑是实现这一目标的关键。

海峡两岸医药卫生交流协会银屑病专业委员会主任委员张晓艳教授、副主任委员刘晓明教授和钟文宏教授等组织皮肤病学专家撰写的《成人寻常型银屑病医患共决策——海峡两岸及港澳地区专家共识》，不仅汇聚了海峡两岸与港澳地区皮肤病学专家建立在循证医学基础上的专业共识和集体智慧，具有较高的学术水平，还参考了海峡两岸与港澳地区银屑病患者代表的意见和建议。

本共识是中国首个银屑病医患共决策专家共识，充分考虑了患者的需求和意愿，内容简明扼要，重点突出，图文并茂，可读性强。相信本共识能为广大的皮肤科医生选择科学的治疗方案提供指导，同时也能为银屑病患者参与诊疗决策提供帮助，有助于提升诊疗质量，提高患者对治疗的依从性和满意度。

本共识的出版充分弘扬了"两岸一家亲，融合向未来"的理念，为推动海峡两岸皮肤病学事业的共同发展做出了贡献！

2024年1月

Foreword

Psoriasis is a chronic, recurrent, inflammatory, and systemic disease, with psoriasis vulgaris being the most common type. In addition to skin lesions, patients with psoriasis are at a significantly increased risk of developing systemic comorbidities such as cardiovascular disease and metabolic diseases, which brings a heavy burden to their physical and mental health, as well as their families and society.

In recent years, with the deepening of research on the pathogenesis of psoriasis and the rapid development of biopharmaceutical technologies, biologic agents and small-molecule targeted drugs have emerged successively, significantly improving the clinical efficacy of patients and their prognosis. However, the recurrence of the disease and the progress of comorbidities have not been effectively controlled, and infections, allergies, secondary unresponsiveness, etc. often occur with treatment. Patients have a low awareness of treatment plans and a low compliance with treatment, which further highlights these issues.

The key to preventing and reducing the aforementioned risks is to choose a reasonable and personalized treatment plan based on the patient's condition, improve the patient's compliance with treatment, and enable them to actively and positively accept scientific and standardized treatment. Effective communication between the doctor and patient, with the doctor playing a leading role in the decision-making process, is undoubtedly the key to achieving this goal.

The *Shared decision-making between physician and patient in adult psoriasis vulgaris-A consensus among experts cross the Straits, Hong Kong and Macao* was written by dermatologists, including Professor Zhang Xiaoyan, the chairman of the Psoriasis Professional Committee of the Cross-Straits Medical and Health Exchange Association; Professor Liu Xiaoming, the vice chairman; and Professor Zhong Wenhong. This consensus not only brings together professional consensus and collective wisdom from dermatologists on both sides of the Taiwan Straits and Hong Kong-Macao region, which is based on evidence-based medicine with a high academic level, but also takes into account the opinions and suggestions of psoriasis patient representatives on both sides of the Taiwan Straits and Hong Kong-Macao region.

The consensus is the first expert consensus on psoriasis in China that emphasizes the needs and wishes of patients, with concise and focused content, vivid graphics, strong readability. It is believed that this consensus can provide guidance for dermatologists to choose scientific treatment plans, while also providing assistance for psoriasis patients to participate in treatment decision-making. This will help improve the quality of diagnosis and treatment, increase patient adherence with treatment and satisfaction.

The publication of this Consensus fully advocates the concept of "Both sides of the Taiwan Straits are one family, integrating towards the futures", and contributes to the common development of cross-strait dermatological services!

Liao Wanping

January 2024

前　言

　　银屑病严重影响患者的身心健康，需要科学防治与长期管理。随着银屑病分子机制研究的深入及新型靶向药物相继问世，越来越多的药物应用于银屑病治疗，医患双方在面临诸多治疗选择时，如何决策将直接影响治疗效果。虽然靶向治疗显著提高了疗效，但也不断出现新的问题和新的瓶颈，需要得到有效解决。医患双方对疾病防治的认知水平都需要不断提升，以提高患者对治疗的依从性和满意度，从而提高疗效和减少复发。

　　为了促进成人寻常型银屑病的规范诊疗，提升皮肤科医生的治疗决策能力，促进和指导医患双方共同参与制订诊疗方案，引导患者加强对银屑病的自身管理，增进诊疗活动中患者的多重获益，由海峡两岸医药卫生交流协会银屑病专业委员会发起，由我及钟文宏、张春雷、刘晓明等银屑病领域知名专家牵头，组织专委会的大陆及港、澳、台专家，共同撰写了《成人寻常型银屑病医患共决策——海峡两岸及港澳地区专家共识》。

　　我们首先设计了患者问卷，下发八个中心对银屑病患者进行问卷调查，收回有效问卷共368份。初步分析结果显示，超过15%的患者不了解自己的病情；近15%的患者对各种治疗方案一无所知；近80%的患者认为自己需要系统治疗，不清楚如何选择；无论传统治疗还是新型靶向药物治疗，患者最关注的都是疗效，尤其是皮损清除率，其次是治疗方案的安全性，此结果与中国患者治疗需求调查结果及国外患者治疗偏好调查结果相似。结合上述调查结果，参考国内外指南及银屑病诊疗与研究进展，聚焦成人寻常型银屑病，充分听取史星翔、柯怡谋、黎庆坤等患者代表的意见和建议，以图文并茂的形式简明扼要地展现寻常型银屑病现有的治疗方法及医患决策流程。各位编者分工撰写，经过十余次线上会议研讨、修改，最后汇总成稿，王丽华老师对全文进行图文编辑，再经过线下与线上的多次审校、修改，形成中英文双语共识终稿。

本共识的宗旨是指导医生和患者共同参与银屑病诊疗决策及疾病的长期管理。

由于时间紧迫，且本共识属于银屑病医患共决策共识的首次尝试，不足之处在所难免，欢迎广大同道提出宝贵意见，编者团队将于再版时加以更新与完善。

2024年1月

Preface

Psoriasis is a disease that seriously affects the physical and mental health of patients. It requires scientific prevention and long–term management. With the continuous deepening of research on the molecular mechanism of psoriasis and the advent of new targeted drugs, more and more drugs have been applied to the treatment of psoriasis, and the treatment goals and methods of psoriasis have also undergone significant changes. When faced with many treatment options, it is particularly important for doctors and patients to make decisions. Although targeted therapies have notably improved efficacy, they also bring forth new challenges and bottlenecks that require effective solutions. The awareness and understanding of disease prevention and management need continual enhancement from both healthcare providers and patients to improve treatment compliance and satisfaction, thereby enhancing efficacy and reducing relapses.

To promote the standardized diagnosis and treatment of adult vulgar psoriasis, enhance the therapeutic decision–making ability of dermatologists, facilitate the joint development of treatment plans between doctors and patients, encourage patients to strengthen their self–management of psoriasis, and enhance multiple benefits for patients in the diagnosis and treatment activities, the Psoriasis Professional Committee of the Cross–Straits Medical and Health Exchange Association initiated the development of *Shared decision–making between physician and patient in adult psoriasis vulgaris – A consensus among experts cross the Straits, Hong Kong and Macao*, which was jointly authored by myself and co–editors Dr. Zhong Wenhong, Dr. Zhang Chunlei, Dr. Liu Xiaoming, and other renowned experts in the field of psoriasis, organized experts from Mainland China, Hong Kong, Macau, and Taiwan.

The editorial committee initially designed a patient questionnaire and distributed it to eight medical centers to conduct a survey on psoriasis patients. A total of 368 valid questionnaires were collected. Preliminary analysis results revealed that more than 15% of the patients did not unaware of their condition, and nearly 15% of the patients knew nothing about various treatment options; nearly 80% of the patients believed that they needed systematic treatment and were not clear about how to choose; regardless of traditional treatment or new targeted drug therapy, the patients were most concerned about the efficacy, especially the clearance rate of skin lesions, followed by the safety of treatment options. This result is similar to the survey results of Chinese patients' treatment needs and foreign patients' treatment preferences. Combining the above survey results with references from domestic and international guidelines, as well as advancements in psoriasis diagnosis, treatment, and research, the focus was on adult plaque psoriasis. The opinions and suggestions of patient representatives such as Shi Xingxiang, Ke Yimou, and Li Qingkun, were fully considered. The existing treatment methods and the medical-patient decision-making process for plaque psoriasis were concisely presented in a visual and informative format. Each editor contributed to the writing, and after more than ten online meetings, discussions, and revisions, the final draft was compiled. Professor Wang Lihua performed graphic and textual editing on the entire manuscript. Following multiple rounds of offline and online proofreading and modifications, the consensus document was finalized in both Chinese and English.

The purpose of this consensus is to guide physicians and patients in jointly participating in psoriasis diagnosis, treatment decisions, and long-term disease management.

Due to time constraints and the fact that this consensus represents the initial attempt at a collaborative agreement between psoriasis healthcare providers and patients, shortcomings are unavoidable. We welcome valuable feedback from our colleagues, and the editorial team will make updates and improvements in subsequent editions.

Xiaoyan Zhong

January 2024

目　录
Contents

第一章

成人寻常型银屑病的诊断与病情评估

一、诊断

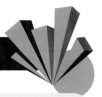

- 皮疹通常表现为慢性反复发作的红色丘疹、斑块，伴多层银白色鳞屑。
- 头皮、四肢伸侧多见，常对称分布，指（趾）甲、黏膜及关节亦可受累。
- 大部分患者症状冬重夏轻，部分患者有家族史。
- 根据典型的临床特点常可明确诊断，临床表现不典型时可通过皮肤镜、组织病理等辅助诊断。

二、病情评估

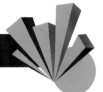

在进行治疗决策前，首先要对病情进行评估。评估指标主要包括：

- 皮损体表面积（body surface area，BSA）
- 银屑病皮损面积及严重程度指数（psoriasis area and severity index，PASI）
- 皮肤病生活质量指数（dermatology life quality index，DLQI）
- 研究者整体评估（investigator's global assessment，IGA）。

通过评估，将病情判定为轻度、中度和重度。具体评分方法见附录A～附录D。

第二章

成人寻常型银屑病医患共决策基本流程

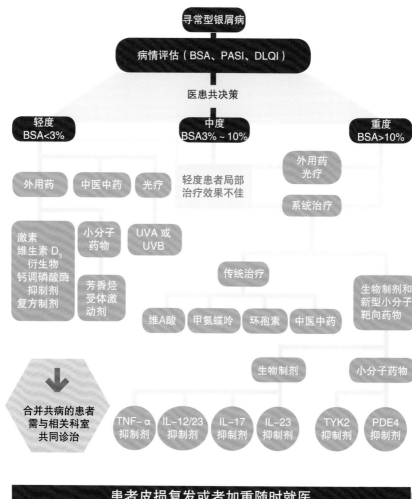

寻常型银屑病

病情评估（BSA、PASI、DLQI）

医患共决策

| 轻度 BSA<3% | 中度 BSA3%~10% | 重度 BSA>10% |

轻度患者局部治疗效果不佳

外用药 光疗

系统治疗

外用药　中医中药　光疗

激素 维生素D₃ 衍生物 钙调磷酸酶抑制剂 复方制剂

小分子药物　芳香烃受体激动剂

UVA 或 UVB

传统治疗

维A酸　甲氨蝶呤　环孢素　中医中药

生物制剂和新型小分子靶向药物

合并共病的患者需与相关科室共同诊治

生物制剂

小分子药物

TNF-α 抑制剂　IL-12/23 抑制剂　IL-17 抑制剂　IL-23 抑制剂　TYK2 抑制剂　PDE4 抑制剂

患者皮损复发或者加重随时就医

评估疗效

医患共决策

医患都满意　维持治疗或者降阶梯　减少系统用药剂量，只用外用药或者光疗

医生或者患者有一方不满意　商讨治疗方案

医患都不满意　更换治疗方案或者升阶梯

升阶梯包括传统用药换为生物制剂或者生物制剂之间的更换，原则为医患共决策，在医生指导下更换，可以换同一靶点的，也可以换不同靶点的生物制剂或小分子药物，也可以转换为传统治疗或联合治疗

第三章

成人寻常型银屑病的治疗方案

一、传统治疗

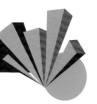

（一）维A酸类

1.作用机制

维A酸（Acitretin）可抑制角质形成细胞增殖，促进表皮角质形成细胞正常分化，同时具有抗炎作用。

2.适应证

中重度寻常型银屑病。

3.用药方案

口服给药，成人起始剂量为20~30mg/d或0.3~0.5mg/（kg·d）。维持剂量则可以基于临床疗效与患者的耐受度进行调整。服用方式最好每日1次，与食物或牛奶一起服用。

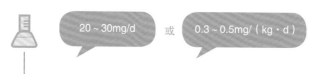

20~30mg/d 或 0.3~0.5mg/（kg·d）

维持剂量则可以基于临床疗效与患者的耐受度进行调整

 服用方式 每日1次，与食物或牛奶一起服用

4.预期疗效

治疗 12 周，PASI 50 和 PASI 75 达标率分别为 20%～70.5%、10%～47%；治疗 24 周，PASI 50 和 PASI 75 达标率分别为 40%～50%、22%～30%。

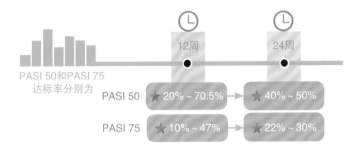

5.常见不良反应

皮肤黏膜干燥、口唇干涩、皮肤变薄、脱屑、甲易脆、甲沟炎，还可能出现血脂升高、肝功能异常、光敏感等。

6.药物间相互作用

避免与四环素类药物、酒精、维生素 A 同时使用。

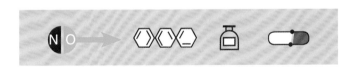

7.禁忌证

（1）此类药有致畸性，孕妇绝对禁用。

（2）有妊娠计划的妇女，在用药前 4 周、用药期间及停药后 2～3 年内避孕。

（3）严重肝肾功能异常、严重高脂血症者禁用。

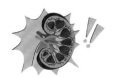

（二）甲氨蝶呤

1.作用机制

甲氨蝶呤（methotrexate，MTX）是一种叶酸拮抗剂，抑制二氢叶酸转变成四氢叶酸，从而抑制DNA合成和细胞增殖。

2.适应证

中、重度寻常型银屑病。

3.用药方案

起始剂量	增加剂量	维持剂量
● 每周2.5~7.5mg，可以口服、皮下注射或肌内注射。 ● 有新上市预充剂型，10mg/支、15mg/支（大陆）。 ● 由于老年人体内叶酸储存下降，肝脏和肾脏功能减退，可考虑小剂量给药，如每周2.5mg。	● 每2~4周增加2.5mg，逐渐增加剂量至每周15~25mg。 ● 常用剂量每周7.5~15mg。	● 病情控制后至少维持1个月后逐渐减量，每4周减2.5mg，直至最小维持量。

★ 近年相关研究显示，与口服MTX相比，皮下注射给药有明确的优势，其生物利用度及疗效更佳，且显著减少胃肠道等不良反应，预充注射剂型使用更加方便。

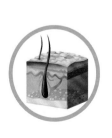
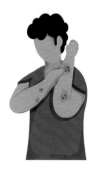

4.预期疗效

治疗16周，PASI 75达标率为36%～41%。

5.常见不良反应

胃肠道反应、肝酶水平升高、骨髓抑制、肝纤维化及甲氨蝶呤诱发的表皮坏死等。

6.药物间相互作用

氨基糖苷类及环孢素等肾毒性药物可减少MTX的肾脏排泄，萘普生、布洛芬等非甾体抗炎药可增强或协同MTX的毒性作用，水杨酸类、磺胺等药物可置换与血浆蛋白结合的MTX，双嘧达莫可增加MTX在细胞内的积累，与维A酸同用可增加肝毒性。

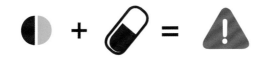

7.禁忌证

妊娠期或哺乳期妇女、骨髓功能障碍及严重感染等。

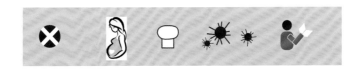

（三）环孢素

1.作用机制

环孢素（Cyclosporin）是一种环状多肽，可选择性抑制T淋巴细胞。

2.适应证

中重度寻常型银屑病。

3.用药方案

（1）常用推荐剂量3～5mg/（kg·d），分2次口服。

（2）推荐起始剂量2.5mg/（kg·d），治疗4周，随后每2周增加0.5mg/（kg·d），至最大剂量5mg/（kg·d）。

（3）若使用耐受最大剂量超过6周后仍无满意疗效，则必须停药。

（4）症状控制后逐渐减量，每2周减0.5～1.0mg/kg，直至最低有效维持剂量。

（5）治疗策略：包括间歇式短程疗法、持续性长程疗法、救援疗法、交替治疗及周末疗法。

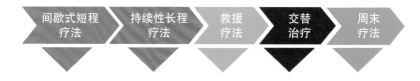

4.预期疗效

环孢素2.5～5.0mg/（kg·d）治疗银屑病16周

PASI 50的应答率为 94% 、PASI 75的应答率为 65% 、PASI 90的应答率为 29% 。

5.常见不良反应

高血压、肾功能异常、震颤、厌食、恶心、呕吐、高血脂、多毛、痤疮等。用药期间须监测血常规、肝肾功能、血脂、血清钾离子和镁离子。

6.药物相互作用

别嘌醇、他汀类、大环内酯类抗生素、抗真菌药等可升高环孢素的血药浓度，抗癫痫药、异烟肼、利福平等药物可降低环孢素的血药浓度，环孢素与他汀类药物同时使用存在横纹肌溶解的风险。

7.禁忌证

肾功能损害、高血压、恶性肿瘤等。

（四）紫外线光疗法

1.作用机制

紫外线光疗法是利用特定波长的紫外线（ultraviolet, UV）治疗疾病的方法。包括长波紫外线（UVA）和中波紫外线（UVB）两种，具有免疫调节及抑制炎症反应的作用。

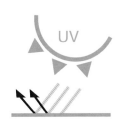

2.适应证

中重度寻常型银屑病。

3.治疗方案

（1）窄谱UVB（narrow band UVB，NB-UVB）：剂量依照患者的肤色或皮肤最小红斑量进行调整。每周治疗2～3次，剂量根据治疗反应逐渐增加。可联合外用药物、系统药物治疗。

（2）UVA（UVA-1，PUVA）：可作为治疗手段之一，但目前较少使用。

（3）308nm准分子光：一种高度选择性的光疗法，用于银屑病局部治疗。

4.预期疗效

NB-UVB治疗4周后，>70%的患者有显著的改善。Meta分析结果显示，NB-UVB治疗PASI 75的达标率为62%。

5.常见不良反应

皮肤干燥、脱屑、发红、色素沉着，严重者可有疼痛、水疱等。

6.禁忌证

（1）绝对禁忌证：伴光敏感的先天性疾病及可能合并或导致皮肤癌的遗传性疾病。

（2）相对禁忌证：光敏感皮肤疾病、黑色素瘤病史、器官移植接受免疫抑制治疗的患者，以及有砷中毒等罹患皮肤癌高风险因素的患者。

7. 其他建议

建议在医生指导下接受治疗，如使用光敏感药物或食物需告知医生。

（五）外用药物

1. 治疗寻常型银屑病外用药物的分类、名称、作用机制及其临床应用（表3-1）。

表3-1　寻常型银屑病外用药物分类、名称、作用机制及其临床应用

分类		名称	作用机制	治疗效果	使用方法	不良反应	禁忌证
糖皮质激素	超强效	0.02%～0.05%丙酸氯倍他索软膏等	抗增生抗炎症免疫抑制	1～2天起效，用药1周后显著改善	每日1～2次；时间<2周，每周<50g	局部：皮肤萎缩、毛细血管扩张、多毛、感染等 全身：下丘脑-垂体-肾上腺轴抑制	药品成分过敏者，皮肤感染、萎缩者
	强效	0.05%卤米松乳膏等					
	中效	0.1%丁酸氢化可的松软膏等					
	弱效	0.05%地奈德乳膏等					
维生素D₃衍生物		0.005%卡泊三醇软膏/搽剂	抗增生促分化免疫调节	1～2周起效，用药4～6周后显著改善	每日2次，间歇使用<1年；持续使用<20周，每周<100g	局部皮肤刺激，可逆性血清钙升高	药品成分过敏者，钙代谢失调者
		0.0002%他卡西醇软膏					
维A酸类药物		0.1%、0.05%他扎罗汀乳膏/凝胶		12周较好疗效/皮损清除	每日1次	局部皮肤刺激，光敏感	药品成分过敏者，妊娠、计划妊娠、哺乳期妇女
钙调磷酸酶抑制剂		1%吡美莫司乳膏	抗炎症免疫调节	2周起效，8周半数以上患者皮损基本消退	每日2次		
		0.03%、0.1%他克莫司软膏					

续　表

分类	名称	作用机制	治疗效果	使用方法	不良反应	禁忌证
角质促成剂	3%水杨酸乳膏、10%尿素乳膏等	促分化	恢复皮肤屏障，辅助治疗	每日1~2次	局部皮肤刺激	药品成分过敏者，5%以上浓度水杨酸不用于妊娠、哺乳期妇女
角质松解剂	5%~10%水杨酸乳膏、20%~40%尿素乳膏等	抗增生去角质				
复方制剂	卡泊三醇倍他米松软膏	抗增生促分化抗炎症免疫抑制免疫调节	1周和4周PASI分别下降39.2%、71.3%	每日1次，持续使用<16周，间歇使用<1年	皮肤刺激、毛细血管扩张、感染、萎缩、高钙血症、肾上腺皮质抑制	药品成分过敏者，钙代谢失调者，皮肤感染、萎缩者
	他扎罗汀倍他米松乳膏		4周有效率65.0%	每日1次，每周用量<45g，疗程4~8周	皮肤刺激、干燥、脱屑、皮肤感染、萎缩、毛细血管扩张，肾上腺皮质抑制	药品成分过敏者，妊娠、计划妊娠、哺乳期妇女，皮肤感染、萎缩者
	复方丙酸氯倍他索软膏		4周痊愈率44.01%，有效率90.52%	每日2次，持续使用不超过4周		

2.外用药物的优化选择和使用原则

（1）根据皮损面积：BSA<3%，可考虑单纯外用药；BSA≥3%，可考虑外用药联合系统治疗、紫外线光疗等。

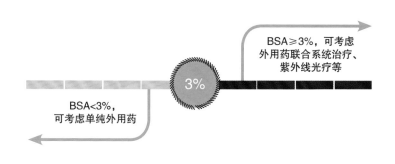

（2）根据皮损部位

面部及皱褶部位：钙调磷酸酶抑制剂、他卡西醇，可短期选择弱/中效激素。

四肢伸侧、臀部、掌跖部位：强/超强效激素、卡泊三醇、他扎罗汀、本维莫德、复方制剂。

头皮部位：糖皮质激素溶液、卡泊三醇搽剂、卡泊三醇倍他米松凝胶。

（3）根据皮损特点：皮损红斑、鳞屑和浸润程度不同，优化选择不同药物种类。

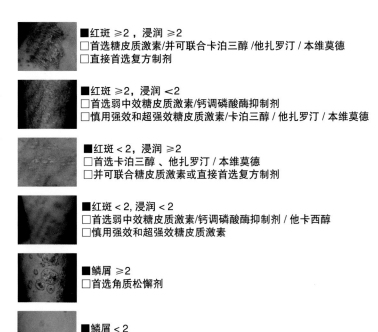

■红斑 ≥2，浸润 ≥2
□首选糖皮质激素/并可联合卡泊三醇/他扎罗汀/本维莫德
□直接首选复方制剂

■红斑 ≥2，浸润 <2
□首选弱中效糖皮质激素/钙调磷酸酶抑制剂
□慎用强效和超强效糖皮质激素/卡泊三醇/他扎罗汀/本维莫德

■红斑 <2，浸润 ≥2
□首选卡泊三醇、他扎罗汀/本维莫德
□并可联合糖皮质激素或直接首选复方制剂

■红斑 <2，浸润 <2
□首选弱中效糖皮质激素/钙调磷酸酶抑制剂/他卡西醇
□慎用强效和超强效糖皮质激素

■鳞屑 ≥2
□首选角质松懈剂

■鳞屑 <2
□首选润肤剂/角质促成剂

注：红斑、浸润及鳞屑具体评估参考附件PASI评分。

（4）外用药物剂量

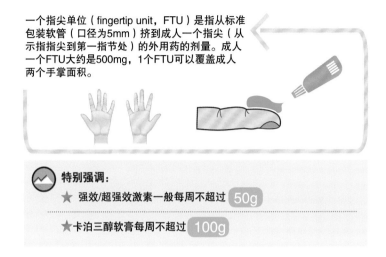

一个指尖单位（fingertip unit，FTU）是指从标准包装软管（口径为5mm）挤成成人一个指尖（从示指指尖到第一指节处）的外用药的剂量。成人一个FTU大约是500mg，1个FTU可以覆盖成人两个手掌面积。

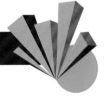

特别强调：

★ 强效/超强效激素一般每周不超过 50g

★卡泊三醇软膏每周不超过 100g

（5）外用药物频率：每日外用1~2次。

（6）封包：适用于局限、顽固、肥厚性皮损，可增加药物渗透，提高疗效。

（7）主动维持治疗：皮损消退后需继续使用润肤剂、角质促成剂等，预防皮损复发。

二、生物制剂及小分子靶向药物

（一）生物制剂

1.概述

目前针对银屑病分子靶点的生物制剂主要包括白介素（interleukin，IL）-17抑制剂、IL-12/23抑制剂和IL-23抑制剂、肿瘤坏死因子α（tumour necrosis factor-α）抑制剂。以下将对生物制剂的机制、适应证、用药前筛查、疗效及安全性等进行简要概述。

2. IL-17A 抑制剂

获批用于治疗成人寻常型银屑病的IL-17A及其受体抑制剂（表3-2）。

表3-2　IL-17A抑制剂的分子特征、适应证、用法、疗效及不良反应

项目		司库奇尤单抗（Secukinumab）	依奇珠单抗（Ixekizumab）	布罗达单抗（Brodalumab）
作用靶点		IL-17A	IL-17A	IL-17RA
分子特征		全人源单克隆抗体	人源化单克隆抗体（98.2%人源+1.8%鼠源）	全人源单克隆抗体
适应证	大陆地区	符合系统治疗或光疗指征的中重度斑块状银屑病6岁及以上患者	符合系统治疗或光疗的中重度斑块状银屑病成人患者	未上市
	台湾地区	符合接受全身性治疗的中重度斑块状银屑病6岁及以上患者	符合接受全身性治疗的中重度斑块状银屑病6岁以上儿童及成人患者	适合接受全身性治疗的中重度斑块状银屑病成人患者
	香港、澳门特别行政区	需要全身性治疗的成人及6岁以上中重度斑块状银屑病患者	需要全身性治疗的中重度斑块状银屑病成人患者	对光疗和其他传统全身疗法反应不足的寻常型银屑病患者及皮疹面积超过10%的患者，顽固性皮损患者
用药方法皮下注射	诱导期	每周1次，每次300mg，连用5次，体重<60kg或>90kg，酌情调整剂量	首次160mg，之后2周1次，每次80mg，连用7次	每周1次，每次210mg，连用3次
	维持期	每4周300mg；体重<60kg，每4周150mg	每4周80mg	每2周210mg

续　表

项目	司库奇尤单抗 （Secukinumab）	依奇珠单抗 （Ixekizumab）	布罗达单抗 （Brodalumab）
预期疗效	12周：PASI 90/100分别为91.7%、39.7%；52周：PASI 90/100分别为91.1%、68.8%；5年：PASI 90/100分别为66.4%、41%	12周：PASI 90/100分别为82.4%、33%；52周：PASI 90/100分别为84%、64%；5年：PASI 90/100分别为67.1%、46.2%	12周：PASI 90/100分别为77.8%、63.3%；52周：PASI 90/100分别为81.8%、72.7%；2.3年：PASI 90/100分别为86%、74%
常见不良反应	鼻炎等上呼吸道感染、单纯疱疹、真菌感染	注射部位反应、咽痛等上呼吸道感染、真菌感染、单纯疱疹	口咽痛等流感症状、注射部位反应、真菌感染
禁忌证	对药物成分过敏、严重的活动性感染（如活动性肺结核）、炎症性肠病等		

3. IL-12/23 抑制剂及 IL-23 抑制剂

获批用于银屑病治疗的 IL-12/23 抑制剂及 IL-23 抑制剂（表3-3）。

表3-3　IL-12/23 及 IL-23 抑制剂的分子特征、适应证、用法、疗效及不良反应

项目		乌司奴单抗 （Ustekinumab）	古塞奇尤单抗 （Guselkumab）	瑞莎珠单抗 （Risankizumab）
作用靶点		IL-12/23 的 p40 亚基	IL-23 的 p19 亚基	IL-23 的 p19 亚基
分子特征		全人源		
适应证	大陆地区	符合接受光疗法或全身性治疗的成人中重度斑块状银屑病	成人中重度寻常型银屑病	中重度寻常型银屑病
	台湾地区			
	香港、澳门特别行政区	6岁及以上中重度斑块状银屑病	符合全身性治疗的成人中重度斑块状银屑病	
用药方法：皮下注射	诱导期	第0、4周，体重≤100kg，每次45mg；体重>100kg，每次90mg	第0、4周各100mg	第0、4周各150mg
	维持期	每12周1次，体重≤100mg，每次45mg；体重>100kg，每次90mg	每8周1次，每次100mg	每12周1次，每次150mg

续　表

项目	乌司奴单抗 （Ustekinumab）	古塞奇尤单抗 （Guselkumab）	瑞莎珠单抗 （Risankizumab）
预期疗效	12～16周：45mg与90mg组，PASI 90/100分别为42%、13%和37%、11% 48～52周：45mg与90mg组，PASI 90分别为58%和71% 5年：PASI 90为60%	16周：PASI 90/100分别为73%、37% 48周：PASI 90/100分别为76.3%、47.4% 5年：PASI 90为82%	16周：PASI 90/100分别为75.3%、35.9% 52周：PASI 90/100分别为82%、56% 172周：PASI 90/100分别为85.5%、54.4%
常见不良反应	上呼吸道感染、头痛等	上呼吸道感染、头痛等	上呼吸道感染、头痛、真菌感染、倦怠等
禁忌证	对药物任何成分过敏，有严重活动性感染等		

4. TNF-α抑制剂

获批用于治疗成人寻常型银屑病的TNF-α治抑制剂（表3-4）。

表3-4　TNF-α抑制剂的分子特征、适应证、用法、疗效及不良反应

项目		阿达木单抗 （Adalimumab）	依那西普 （Etanercept）	英夫利昔单抗 （Infliximab）
作用靶点		TNF-i	TNF-i	TNF-i
分子特征		重组全人源单克隆抗体	人源化TNF-源受体-抗体融合蛋白	人-鼠嵌合型单克隆抗体
适应证	大陆地区	需要系统治疗的成人中重度斑块状银屑病；≥4岁儿童重度斑块状银屑病	成人中重度斑块状银屑病	需要系统治疗，但传统系统药物或光疗无效、禁忌或不耐受的成人中重度斑块状银屑病
	台湾地区	其他全身性治疗或光疗无效、有禁忌或无法耐受的中重度银屑病成人患者	—	
	香港、澳门特别行政区	成人中重度斑块状银屑病		

续　表

项目		阿达木单抗 （Adalimumab）	依那西普 （Etanercept）	英夫利昔单抗 （Infliximab）
用药方法	诱导期	皮下注射，初始剂量80mg，第2周40mg	皮下注射，25mg/次，每周2次；或50mg/次，每周1次	静脉滴注，第0、2、6周予5mg/kg
	维持期	皮下注射，每2周40mg		静脉滴注，每隔8周给药1次，每次5mg/kg
预期疗效		12周：PASI 75/90分别为58.7%~77.8%、30.43% 52周：PASI 75/90分别为73.3%、60.4% 160周：PASI 75/90分别为76%、50%	12周：PASI 75/90分别为40.98%、21% 24周：PASI 75为66.3% 3年：PASI 75为88.2%	10周：PASI 75/90分别为81%、57.1%
常见不良反应		上呼吸道感染、注射部位反应、狼疮样综合征等	上呼吸道感染、注射部位反应、头痛等	上呼吸道感染、输液反应、血清病样反应、充血性心力衰竭等
禁忌证		对药物成分过敏者、活动性肺结核等活动性感染、中重度充血性心力衰竭、病情尚未有效控制的恶性肿瘤		

5.筛查和监测

生物制剂用药前筛查及用药期间监测指标（表3-5）。

表3-5　生物制剂用药前筛查及监测指标

检查项目	用药前	用药期间
血常规、尿常规和肝功能	√	用药第4、12周及以后每3个月检查1次
肾功能	√	无特殊要求
乙肝、丙肝血清学检测	√	筛查阳性者根据情况每3~6个月检查1次
HIV血清学检测	根据患者情况而定	无特殊要求
抗核抗体	TNF-α抑制剂	TNF-α抑制剂每半年检查1次
结核筛查（PPD或T-SPOT或QuantiFERON-TB Gold）	√	TNF-α抑制剂每半年检查1次，其他生物制剂每年检查1次

续　表

检查项目	用药前	用药期间
胸部X线或CT检查	√	TNF-α抑制剂每半年检查1次，其他生物制剂每年检查1次
肿瘤筛查	根据患者情况而定	无特殊要求

注：HIV，人类免疫缺陷病毒；T-SPOT，T细胞斑点检测；TNF-α，肿瘤坏死因子α；PPD，结核菌素纯蛋白衍生物试验。

6.特殊人群生物制剂用药建议（表3-6）。

表3-6　特殊人群生物制剂用药建议

特殊人群	用药建议
妊娠期与哺乳期	权衡利弊，必要时谨慎选择使用
结核病患者	活动性结核禁用TNF-α制剂；非活动性结核病和结核分枝杆菌潜伏感染患者，感染科会诊，决定是否预防性抗结核治疗
HBV感染者	必要时须检测血中HBV-DNA定量、监测肝功能，一旦发现HBV再激活，按HBV活动性感染处理，感染科诊治
恶性肿瘤者	活动期肿瘤禁用，治疗后稳定≥5年的肿瘤患者可以应用；须严密监测，权衡利弊后考虑是否给药
手术患者	中高风险手术，停用生物制剂3~5个半衰期后再进行择期手术；低风险手术患者生物制剂的使用不受影响
疫苗接种	成人用药期间避免接种活疫苗；妊娠16周之后使用生物制剂者，其分娩的婴儿出生后6个月内避免接种活疫苗
炎性肠病患者	不适合选择IL-17A抑制剂
其他特殊人群	咨询医生

（二）小分子靶向药物

1.阿普米司特

（1）作用机制：阿普米司特（Apremilast）可特异性地抑制磷酸二酯酶4（phosphodiesterase，PDE4），阻断环磷酸腺苷降解，进而抑制促炎因子的合成和释放。

（2）适应证：全球首个获批靶向PDE4的治疗银屑病的小分子口服药物，中国大陆获批用于治疗符合光疗或系统治疗指征的成人中重度斑块状银屑病。

（3）用药方案

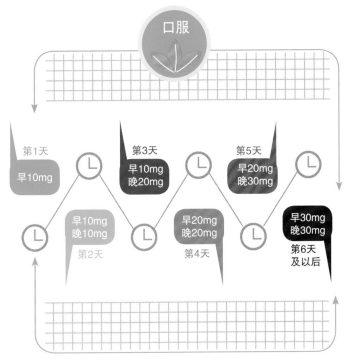

（4）预期疗效：治疗16周、32周和52周，PASI 75达标率分别为33.1%、35%和61%。

（5）常见不良反应：腹泻、恶心和呕吐等，大部分为轻中度，常发生在用药前2周，多数在1个月内缓解。如发生不明原因的体重下降，应进行评估，必要时考虑停用本品。

（6）药物间相互作用：不建议与利福平、苯巴比妥、卡马西平、苯妥英钠等药物联合使用。

（7）禁忌证：对阿普米司特或制剂中任何辅料过敏者禁用。存在抑郁和/或自杀想法或行为病史的患者，须权衡风险和获益。

2.氘可来昔替尼

（1）作用机制：氘可来昔替尼（Deucravacitinib）是酪氨酸激酶2

（tyrosine-protein kinase 2，TYK2）变构抑制剂，通过抑制 IL-23/IL-17 介导的免疫炎症治疗银屑病。

（2）适应证：适合系统治疗或光疗的成人中重度斑块状银屑病。

（3）用法用量：口服给药，每日 1 片（6mg）。

（4）预期疗效：治疗 16 周，PASI 75 达标率为 68.8%，头皮特异性临床医师整体评估（scalp-specific physician's global assessment，ss-PGA）0/1 达标率为 64%；52 周，PASI 75/90 达标率分别为 71.0%、45.5%，持久应答，疗效稳定，未衰减。

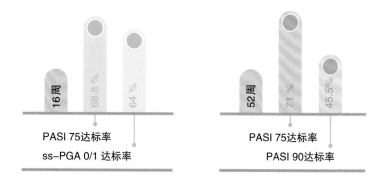

16周 68.8% 64%

PASI 75达标率
ss-PGA 0/1 达标率

52周 71% 45.5%

PASI 75达标率
PASI 90达标率

（5）常见不良反应：鼻咽炎等上呼吸道感染、头痛、腹泻和恶心等。

（6）禁忌证：对本品中任何成分过敏者禁用，活动性感染和恶性肿瘤者禁用。

3.本维莫德乳膏

（1）作用机制：本维莫德（Benverimod）靶向激活芳香烃受体，有效调控相关免疫细胞和炎症因子的表达，直接作用于角质形成细胞，同时抑制新生血管生成和毛细血管扩张。

（2）适应证：适合局部治疗的成人轻中度稳定性寻常型银屑病。

（3）用法用量：早晚各 1 次外用，不建议用于头面部及腹股沟、肛门等皱褶部位。每日最大剂量为 6g，治疗面积小于体表面积的 10%。涂药部位避免紫外线照射。

（4）预期疗效：治疗 12 周，PASI 75 达标率为 50.4%。

（5）常见不良反应：用药部位红肿、瘙痒、接触性皮炎、毛囊炎、色素异常等，多为一过性并呈轻中度，多可自行好转。

（6）药物间相互作用：尚不明确。

（7）禁忌证：对本品中任何成分过敏者禁用；妊娠、计划妊娠及哺乳期妇女禁用；红皮病型银屑病、泛发性脓疱型银屑病等禁用。

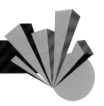

三、中医中药

（一）病因病机

银屑病，中医称之为"白疕"，是由素体内热、外感、情志内伤、饮食失节等导致气机不畅，郁久化热，热毒蕴于血分；病久或反复发作，阴血被耗，化燥生风；或经脉阻滞，气血凝结，肌肤失养所致。

（二）主要辨证分型

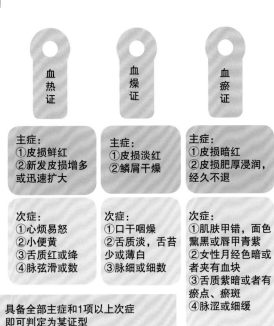

血热证

主症：
①皮损鲜红
②新发皮损增多或迅速扩大

次症：
①心烦易怒
②小便黄
③舌质红或绛
④脉弦滑或数

血燥证

主症：
①皮损淡红
②鳞屑干燥

次症：
①口干咽燥
②舌质淡，舌苔少或薄白
③脉细或细数

血瘀证

主症：
①皮损暗红
②皮损肥厚浸润，经久不退

次症：
①肌肤甲错，面色黧黑或唇甲青紫
②女性月经色暗或者夹有血块
③舌质紫暗或者有瘀点、瘀斑
④脉涩或细缓

判定标准　具备全部主症和1项以上次症即可判定为某证型

（三）辨证论治

不同证型其治则、治法、方药不同。

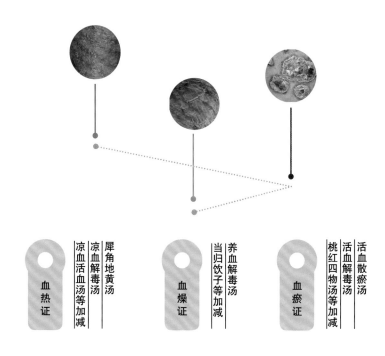

血热证	血燥证	血瘀证
犀角地黄汤 凉血解毒汤 凉血活血汤等加减	养血解毒汤 当归饮子等加减	活血散瘀汤 活血解毒汤 桃红四物汤等加减

（四）口服中成药

血热证	血燥证	血瘀证
复方青黛类 （胶囊、丸、片） 消银类（颗粒、胶囊、片） 银屑胶囊、克银丸 百癣夏塔热片等	消银类（颗粒、胶囊、片） 紫丹银屑胶囊 润燥止痒胶囊等	郁金银屑片 银屑胶囊等

4.注意事项

（1）对本类药品过敏者禁用。

（2）儿童、老人、孕妇、哺乳期妇女慎用。

（3）苦寒药物要注意疗程，避免伤及脾胃。

（4）服药期间，忌烟酒及辛辣油腻、刺激或致敏食物。

5.不良反应

腹泻、腹痛、恶心、呕吐，偶有皮疹瘙痒等。

（五）中医外治法及非药物疗法

根据辨证分型，可针对性给予患者药浴、塌渍、熏蒸、涂擦及封包等中医外治法，以及留罐、闪罐、走罐、刺络拔罐、针刺、穴位埋线、火针、艾灸、三棱针、耳穴等非药物疗法。中医治法手段丰富，灵活度高，无毒副作用，可提高疗效，延缓疾病复发。

（六）中医调护

合理膳食，不盲目忌口，超重或肥胖者应节食减重。忌烟限酒。规律作息，保持良好情绪。康复期遵循"春夏养阳，秋冬养阴"原则。练习八段锦、五禽戏等舒缓身体。在初愈康复阶段，适当采用养血、滋阴、调理脾胃药物巩固疗效。远离六淫疫气，做好皮损消除后的调理与摄养。

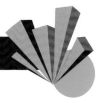

四、银屑病治疗药物作用机制图

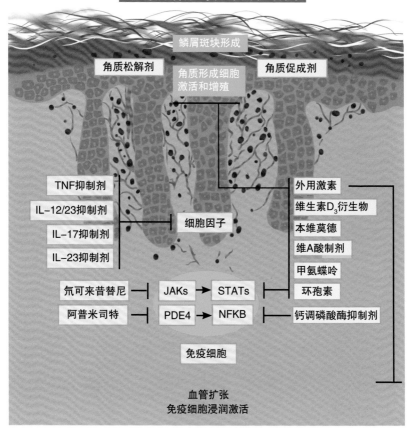

银屑病治疗药物作用机制图

第四章

患者对决策基本过程的知晓情况测试

1. 您认为您的银屑病严重程度如何？（单选）

□轻度　□中度　□重度

2. 您确定选择哪种治疗方法了吗？（不定项选择）

（　）外用药

（　）传统药物系统：□甲氨蝶呤　□环孢素　□维A酸

（　）中医中药

（　）光疗

（　）生物制剂：□司库奇尤单抗　□依奇珠单抗

　　　　　　　　□古塞奇尤单抗　□阿达木单抗

　　　　　　　　□英夫利息单抗　□瑞莎珠单抗

　　　　　　　　□其他

（　）小分子药物：□阿普米司特　□氘可来昔替尼　□本维莫德

（　）我想再考虑一下

3. 如果在治疗过程中您的病情加重，您会选择以下哪种处理方式？（单选）

□自行把药物加量使用

□借鉴病友的治疗经验

□到医院就诊，在医生指导下调整治疗方案

4. 应用生物制剂治疗有哪些重要的注意事项？（多选）

□用药前要严格筛查

□用药期间要定期进行药物安全监测

□用药剂量及间隔时间的调整需要在医生的指导下进行

□皮疹消退可以自行停药

附录 A

体表面积（BSA）评分

　　将患者单个手掌及手指屈侧面积定义为人体表面积的1%，评估患者全身皮损总和达到多少个手掌面积，记为BSA。评估时请参考以下比例：

　　头颈=10%体表面积（10个手掌）

　　上肢=20%体表面积（20个手掌）

　　躯干（含腋窝和腹股沟）=30%体表面积（30个手掌）

　　下肢（含臀部）=40%体表面积（40个手掌）

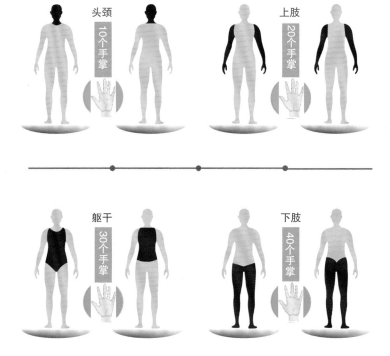

附录B
银屑病皮损面积及严重程度指数（PASI）评分

PASI评分标准包括皮损面积评分和皮损严重程度评分。PASI是评判银屑病病情严重程度的重要指标，也是对银屑病病情轻重进行量化的一个指标，以具体的数字反映银屑病的病情。分值为0~72分，分数越高说明病变范围大，皮损严重（图B-1）。

银屑病皮损严重程度				
0=无皮损，1=轻度，2=中度，3=重度，4=极重度				
	头部	躯干	上肢	下肢
红斑	0~4	0~4	0~4	0~4
浸润	0~4	0~4	0~4	0~4
鳞屑	0~4	0~4	0~4	0~4
合计①	以上分值之和	以上分值之和	以上分值之和	以上分值之和
银屑病皮损受累面积				
0=无皮疹，1<10%，2=10%~29%，3=30%~49%，4=50%~69%，5=70%~89%，6=90%~100%				
受累面积分值②	0~6	0~6	0~6	0~6
①×②乘积	①×②	①×②	①×②	①×②
躯体部位系数	0.1	0.3	0.2	0.4
①×②×③	A	B	C	D
PASI=A+B+C+D （0~72）				

图B-1 银屑病皮损面积及严重程度指数评分

附录C
皮肤病生活质量指数（DLQI）问卷

DLQI评分是银屑病患者生活质量评分，主要是通过问卷调查，了解银屑病对患者日常生活的影响。

DLQI问卷共有10个问题，每个问题有4个不同答案，分别为无、轻微、严重、极严重，对应的分值为0分、1分、2分、3分，最后将10个分值相加，得出总DLQI评分值（程度分级：0~1分，无影响；2~5分，轻度；6~10分，中度；>10分，重度）。

皮肤病生活质量指数问卷

以下问题是为了了解在过去的1周内，皮肤问题对您的生活带来多大的影响。

1. 上周内，您的皮肤感到痒、触痛、疼痛、刺痛了吗？　　□非常多 □许多 □一点 □全没有

2. 上周内，由于您的皮肤问题，您感到尴尬或自卑吗？　　□非常多 □许多 □一点 □全没有

3. 上周内，因为皮肤问题，对您购物、做家务、整理庭院影响程度如何？　　□非常多 □许多 □一点 □全没有

4. 上周内，皮肤问题对您穿衣服影响程度如何？　　□非常多 □许多 □一点 □全没有

5. 上周内，皮肤问题对您的社交或休闲生活有多大的影响？　　□非常多 □许多 □一点 □全没有

6. 上周内，皮肤问题对您运动有多大妨碍？　　□非常多 □许多 □一点 □全没有

7. 上周内，皮肤问题是否妨碍您的上班或学习？　　□非常多 □许多 □一点 □全没有

8. 上周内，皮肤问题妨碍了您和爱人、亲密的朋友、亲戚间的交往了吗？　　□非常多 □许多 □一点 □全没有

9. 上周内，皮肤问题给您的性生活造成了多大影响？　　□非常多 □许多 □一点 □全没有

10. 上周内，由于治疗您的皮肤问题，给您造成了多少麻烦，如把家里弄得一团糟或占用了您很多时间？　　□非常多 □许多 □一点 □全没有

附录 D

研究者整体评估（IGA）

IGA 是皮肤病临床研究中最常用的评估指标之一，用于评估患者病情的严重程度和治疗效果。这种评估方法可以帮助医生和研究者更好地评估患者的整体病情和疗效，并提供定量化的评估结果（表D-1）。

表D-1　研究者整体评估

评分（分）	简短描述	详细描述
0	消退	无银屑病症状，可能存在炎症后色素沉着
1	几乎消退	正常至粉红色皮损，未增厚，没有或极轻微的灶性鳞屑
2	轻度	粉红色至淡红色皮损，可检测到轻度增厚，轻度鳞屑
3	中度	暗亮红色，清楚可辨的红斑，清楚可辨至中度增厚，中等鳞屑
4	重度	亮至深暗红色，重度增厚伴有坚硬的边缘，几乎全部或全部皮损都覆盖有重度/粗的鳞屑

附录 E

中英文对照

中文	英文
维A酸	Acitretin
阿达木单抗	Adalimumab
体表面积	body surface area，BSA
布罗达单抗	Brodalumab
环孢素	Cyclosporin
皮肤病生活质量指数	dermatology life quality index，DLQI
氘可来昔替尼	Deucravacitinib
依那西普	Etanercept
指尖单位	fingertip unit，FTU
古塞奇尤单抗	Guselkumab
英夫利昔单抗	Infliximab
白介素	interleukin，IL
研究者整体评估	investigator's global assessment，IGA
依奇珠单抗	Ixekizumab
甲氨蝶呤	Methotrexate，MTX
窄谱中波紫外线	narrow band UVB，NB-UVB
磷酸二酯酶4	phosphodiesterase，PDE4
银屑病皮损面积及严重程度指数	psoriasis area severity index，PASI
瑞莎珠单抗	Risankizumab
司库奇尤单抗	Secukinumab
头皮特异性临床医师整体评估	scalp-specific physician's global assessment, ss-PGA
肿瘤坏死因子α	tumour necrosis factor-α，TNF-α
紫外线	ultraviolet，UV
乌司奴单抗	Ustekinumab

参 考 文 献

1.陈小兰, 郑丽英, 张昊, 等.银屑病患者疾病负担和生存质量调查: 基于网络的问卷调查 [J].中华皮肤科杂志, 2019, 52(11): 791-795.

2.中华医学会皮肤性病学分会银屑病专业委员会.中国银屑病诊疗指南(2023版)[J].中华 皮肤科杂志, 2023, 56(7): 573-625.

3.中华医学会皮肤性病学分会银屑病学组.本维莫德乳膏治疗银屑病专家指导意见[J].中 国皮肤性病学杂志, 2021, 35(6): 707-711.

4.赵炳南, 张志礼.简明中医皮肤病学[M].北京: 中国中医药出版社, 2014: 190.

5.中华中医药学会皮肤科分会.皮肤科分会银屑病中医治疗专家共识(2017年版)[J]. 中国 中西医结合皮肤性病学杂志, 2018, 17(3): 273-277.

6.陈朝霞, 李萍, 张广中, 等.艾灸治疗血瘀证斑块型银屑病: 随机对照研究[J].中国针灸, 2021, 41(7): 762-766.

7.KOMINE M, KIM H, YI J, et al. A discrete choice experiment on oral and injection treatment preferences among moderate-to-severe psoriasis patients in Japan[J]. J Dermatol, 2023, 50 (6): 766-777.

8.LEE JH, YOUN JI, KIM TY, et al. A multicenter, randomized, open-label pilot trial assessing the efficacy and safety of etanercept 50 mg twice weekly followed by etanercept 25 mg twice weekly, the combination of etanercept 25 mg twice weekly and acitretin, and acitretin alone in patients with moderate to severe psoriasis[J]. BMC Dermatol, 2016, 16 (1): 11.

9.DOGRA S, JAIN A, KANWAR AJ. Efficacy and safety of acitretin in three fixed doses of 25, 35 and 50 mg in adult patients with severe plaque type psoriasis: a randomized, double blind, parallel group, dose ranging study[J]. J Eur Acad Dermatol Venereol, 2013, 27: e305-311.

10.YU C, FAN X, LI Z, et al. Efficacy and safety of total glucosides of paeony combined with acitretin in the treatment of moderate-to-severe plaque psoriasis: a double-blind, ran-domised, placebo-controlled trial[J]. Eur J Dermatol, 2017, 27: 150-154.

11.WARREN RB, MROWIETZ U, VON KIEDROWSKI R, et al. An intensified dosing sched-ule of subcutaneous methotrexate in patients with moderate to severe plaque-type psoriasis (METOP): a 52 week, multicentre, randomised, double-blind, placebo-controlled, phase 3 trial[J]. Lancet, 2017, 389(10068): 528-537.

12.CHEN TJ, CHUNG WH, CHEN CB, et al. Methotrexate-induced epidermal necrosis: A case series of 24 patients[J]. J Am Acad Dermatol, 2017, 77(2): 247-255.

13.RICHARDS HL, FORTUNE DG, O'SULLIVAN TM, et al. Patients with psoriasis and their compliance with medication[J]. J Am Acad Dermatol, 1999, 41(4): 581-583.

14.HO VC, GRIFFITHS CE, BERTH-JONES J, et al. Intermittent short courses of cyclosporine microemulsion for the long-term management of psoriasis: a 2-year cohort study[J]. J Am Acad Dermatol, 2001, 44 (4): 643-651.

15.ELMETS CA, LIM HW, STOFF B, et al. Joint American Academy of Dermatology-National Psoriasis Foundation guidelines of care for the management and treatment of psoriasis with phototherapy[J]. J Am Acad Dermatol, 2019, 81(3): 775-804.

16.GOULDEN V, LING TC, BABAKINEJAD P, et al. British Association of Dermatologistsapy. J Am Acad Dermatol. 2019;81(3): 775-8ation of Dermatologists and British Photodermatology Group guidelines for narrowband ultraviolet B phototherapy 2022[J]. Br J Dermatol, 2022, 187(3): 295-308.

17.DANIEL BS, ORCHARD D. Ocular side-effects of topical corticosteroids: what a dermatologist needs to know[J]. Australas J Dermatol, 2015, 56(3): 164-169.

18.SMITH SH, JAYAWICKREME C, RICKARD DJ, et al. Tapinarof Is a Natural AhR Agonist that Resolves Skin Inflammation in Mice and Humans[J]. J Invest Dermatol, 2017, 137(10): 2110-2119.

19.ZHOU J, YUAN Y, LIU Y, et al. Effectiveness and safety of secukinumab in Chinese patients with moderate to severe plaque psoriasis in real-world practice[J]. Exp Dermatol, 2023. doi: 10.1111/exd.14890.

20.LI XIA, ZHENG JIE, PAN WEI-LI, et al. Efficacy and Safety of Ixekizumab in Chinese Patients with Moderate-to-Severe Plaque Psoriasis: 60-Week Results From a Phase 3 Study [J]. International journal of Dermatology and Venereology, 2022, 5(4): 181-190.

21.BLAUVELT A, LEBWOHL MG, MABUCHI T, et al. Long-term efficacy and safety of ixekizumab: A 5-year analysis of the UNCOVER-3 randomized controlled trial[J]. J Am Acad Dermatol, 2021, 85(2): 360-368.

22.GALLUZZO M, CALDAROLA G, SIMONE CD, et al. Use of brodalumab for the treatment of chronic plaque psoriasis: a one-year real-life study in the Lazio region, Italy[J]. Expert Opin Biol Ther, 2021, 21(9): 1299-1310.

23.LEONARDI CL, KIMBALL AB, PAPP KA, et al. Efficacy and safety of ustekinumab, a human interleukin-12/23 monoclonal antibody, in patients with psoriasis: 76-week results from a randomised, double-blind, placebo-controlled trial (PHOENIX 1) [J]. Lancet, 2008, 371(9625): 1665-1674.

24.PAPP KA, GRIFFITHS CE, GORDON K, et al. Long-term safety of ustekinumab in patients with moderate-to-severe psoriasis: final results from 5 years of follow-up[J]. Br J Dermatol, 2013, 168(4): 844-854.

25.BLAUVELT A, PAPP KA, GRIFFITHS CEM, et al. Efficacy and safety of guselkumab, an anti-interleukin-23 monoclonal antibody, compared with adalimumab for the continuous treatment of patients with moderate to severe psoriasis: Results from the phase III, double-blinded, placebo- and active comparator-controlled VOYAGE 1 trial[J]. J Am Acad Dermatol, 2017, 76(3): 405-417.

26.GORDON KB, STROBER B, LEBWOHL M, et al. Efficacy and safety of risankizumab in moderate-to-severe plaque psoriasis (UltIMMa-1 and UltIMMa-2): results from two double-blind, randomised, placebo-controlled and ustekinumab-controlled phase 3 trials [J]. Lancet, 2018, 392(10148): 650-661.

27.LI GJ, GU YX, ZOU Q, et al. Efficacy, Safety, and Pharmacoeconomic Analysis of Adalimumab and Secukinumab for Moderate-to-Severe Plaque Psoriasis: A Single-Center, Real-World Study[J].Dermatol Ther, 2022, 12(9): 2105-2115.

28.XIE F, WANG R, ZHAO ZG, et al. Safety and efficacy of etanercept monotherapy for moderate-to-severe plaque psoriasis: A prospective 12-week follow-up study[J]. Journal of Huazhong University of Science and Technology, 2017, 37(6): 943-947.

29.PAUL C, CATHER J, GOODERHAM M, et al. Efficacy and safety of apremilast, an oral phosphodiesterase 4 inhibitor, in patients with moderate-to-severe plaque psoriasis over 52 weeks: a phase III, randomized controlled trial(ESTEEM 2)[J]. Br J Dermatol, 2015, 173(6): 1387-1399.

30.ARMSTRONG AW, GOODERHAM M, WARREN RB, et al. Deucravacitinib versus placebo and apremilast in moderate to severe plaque psoriasis: efficacy and safety results from the 52-week, randomized, double-blinded, placebo-controlled phase 3 POETYK PSO-1 trial[J]. J Am Acad Dermatol, 2023, 88(1): 29-39.

31.CAI L, CHEN GH, LU QJ, et al. A double-blind, randomized, placebo- and positive-controlled phase III trial of 1% benvitimod cream in mild-to-moderate plaque psoriasis[J]. Chin Med J, 2020, 133(24): 2905-2909.

致　　谢

　　本共识是海峡两岸及港澳地区皮肤病学专家集体智慧的结晶，廖万清院士欣然为本共识作序，充分体现了学界前辈对本共识的大力支持和高度认可。

　　台湾干癣协会主席柯怡谋先生、香港银友会会长黎庆坤先生、大陆银屑病病友互助网发起人史星翔先生、台湾干癣协会秘书长王雅馨女士等银屑病患者代表对共识的内容也提出了宝贵的意见和建议，使医患共决策的宗旨实至名归。

　　本共识图文并茂的表现形式得益于王丽华老师的辛勤付出。

　　本共识得到了海峡两岸医药卫生交流协会银屑病专业委员会全体委员的关注和支持，海峡两岸医药卫生交流协会领导对本共识的成功出版给予了大力支持和指导。

　　上海市皮肤病医院高芸露医生、鄂尔多斯市中心医院皮肤科郭利平医生、北京大学第三医院皮肤科王晓宇医生也对本共识的写作和翻译提供了大力支持和协助。

　　在此，对给予本共识提供帮助的所有领导、同仁和朋友表示最衷心的感谢！

Chapter1

Diagnosis and Disease Assessment of Adult Psoriasis Vulgaris

Diagnosis

- The rash usually presents as chronic recurrent red papules and plaques with multiple layers of silvery white scales.
- It is more common on the scalp and limb extensor sides, often symmetrically distributed. Nail, mucosa, and joints can also be involved.
- Most cases are severe in winter and mild in summer, and some patients have a family history.
- Diagnosis can often be clearly confirmed based on typical clinical characteristics. When the clinical presentation is atypical, auxiliary diagnosis can be performed through dermoscopy, histopathology, etc.

Evaluation of the Patient's Condition

Before making treatment decisions, it is important to assess the patient's condition first. The evaluation methods which are used to determine the severity of the condition as mild, moderate, or severe mainly include:

- Body surface area (BSA)
- Psoriasis area and severity index (PASI)
- Dermatology life quality index (DLQI)
- Investigator's global assessment (IGA)

The specific scoring methods are shown in Appendix A–Appendix D.

Chapter 2

The Basic Process of Doctor-patient Shared

Decision-making for Adult Psoriasis Vulgaris

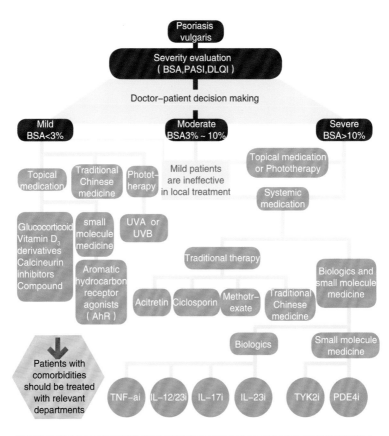

Psoriasis vulgaris

Severity evaluation (BSA,PASI,DLQI)

Doctor—patient decision making

Mild BSA<3%

Moderate BSA3% ~ 10%

Severe BSA>10%

Topical medication

Traditional Chinese medicine

Photot-herapy

Mild patients are ineffective in local treatment

Topical medication or Phototherapy

Systemic medication

Glucocorticoid Vitamin D₃ derivatives Calcineurin inhibitors Compound

small molecule medicine

UVA or UVB

Aromatic hydrocarbon receptor agonists (AhR)

Traditional therapy

Acitretin

Ciclosporin

Methotr-exate

Traditional Chinese medicine

Biologics and small molecule medicine

Patients with comorbidities should be treated with relevant departments

Biologics

Small molecule medicine

TNF–ai

IL–12/23i

IL–17i

IL–23i

TYK2i

PDE4i

Patients with recurrence or aggravation of skin lesions should seek medical attention in time

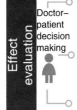

Effect evaluation

Doctor–patient decision making

Both doctors and patients are satisfied

Maintenance treatment or deescaiation therapy

Reduce the dose of systemic medication, or only topical or phototherapy

Neither the doctor nor the patient is satisfied

Discuss treatment

Doctors and patients were not satisfied

Alternative treatment or step–up therapy

The step-up therapy includes the replacement of traditional therapy to biologics or conversion between biologics. The principle is doctor–patient co–decision, under the guidance of doctors, therapeutic regimen can be replaced by the same target or different targets of biologics or small moecule drugs, can also be converted to traditional therapy or combination therapy.

Chapter 3

Treatment of Adult Psoriasis Vulgaris

Traditional Treatment

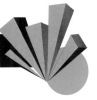

Retinoids

Mechanism of action

Acitretin can inhibit the proliferation of keratinocytes and promote the normal differentiation of epidermal keratinocytes, as well as anti–inflammatory effects.

Indications

Moderate to severe psoriasis vulgaris.

BSA 3%

Therapeutic schedule

The initial dose for adults is 20~30mg/d, or 0.3~0.5mg/(kg·d). The maintenance dose can be adjusted based on clinical efficacy and patient tolerance. It is recommended to be taken once daily, preferably with food or milk.

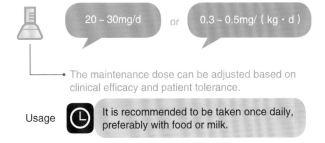

20 ~ 30mg/d　or　0.3 ~ 0.5mg/ (kg · d)

The maintenance dose can be adjusted based on clinical efficacy and patient tolerance.

Usage　It is recommended to be taken once daily, preferably with food or milk.

Expected therapeutic effect

At 12 weeks of treatment, the PASI 50 and PASI 75 response rates are approximately 20%~70.5% and 10%~47%, respectively; After 24 weeks of treatment, the PASI 50 and PASI 75 response rates are around 40%~50% and 22%~30%, respectively.

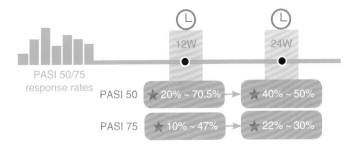

Common adverse reactions

Dry skin and mucous membrane, dry lips, thinning of the skin, desquamation, brittle nails, onychomycosis, elevated blood lipids, liver function abnormalities, photosensitivity, etc. may also occur.

Drug interactions

Avoid concurrent use with tetracycline antibiotics, alcohol, and vitamin A supplements.

Contraindications

This medication is teratogenic and is absolutely contraindicated in pregnant women.

Women planning pregnancy should use contraception 4 weeks before starting the medication, during its use, and for 2~3 years after discontinuation.

It is also contraindicated in individuals with severe liver or kidney dysfunction and severe hyperlipidemia.

Methotrexate（MTX）

Mechanism of action

MTX is a folate antagonist that inhibits the conversion of dihydrofolate to tetrahydrofolate, thereby inhibiting DNA synthesis and cell proliferation.

Indications

Moderate to severe psoriasis vulgaris.

Therapeutic schedule

Initial dosage	Dosage titration	Maintenance dosage
● 2.5~7.5mg once weekly, which can be given orally, subcutaneously or intramuscularly. ● New pre-filled dosage form, 1omg/branch, 15mg/branch (Mainland) ● Due to decreased folate storage and reduced liver and kidney function in the elderly, low-dose administration, such as 2.5mg/ week, may be considered.	● The dose was increased by 2.5mg every 2 to 4 weeks, gradually reaching to 15~25mg/week, and the usual dose was 7.5 to 15mg/week.	● After the disease was controlled for at least 1 months, the dose was gradually reduced by 2.5mg every 4 weeks until the minimum maintenance dose.

★ In recent years, several studies have shown that subcutaneous injection of MTX offers significant advantages over oral intake, for its improved bioavailability and efficacy. It also significantly reduces gastriointestinal reations, and the prefilled injection formulation is more convenient to use.

Expected therapeutic effect

After 16 weeks of treatment, the PASI 75 response rate was 36%~41%.

Common adverse reactions

Gastrointestinal reactions, elevated liver enzymes, bone marrow suppression, liver fibrosis and methotrexate induced epidermal necrosis.

Drug interactions

Nephrotoxic drugs such as aminoglycosides and cyclosporine can reduce the renal excretion of MTX. Naproxen, ibuprofen and other non-steroidal anti-inflammatory drugs can enhance or synergize the toxic effect of MTX. Salicylic acids, sulfonamides and other drugs can displace MTX bound to plasma proteins. Dipyridamole could increase the intracellular accumulation of MTX. Co-administration with tretinoin may increase hepatotoxicity.

Contraindications

Pregnant or lactating women, bone marrow dysfunction and severe infections.

Cyclosporin

Mechanism of action

Cyclosporine is a cyclic peptide that selectively inhibits T lymphocytes.

Indications

Moderate to severe psoriasis vulgaris.

Therapeutic schedule

The recommended dose is 3~5mg /(kg·d), twice a day.

The recommended starting dose is 2.5mg / kg·d for 4 weeks, followed by an increase of 0.5mg / (kg·d) every 2 weeks to the maximum dose of 5mg/(kg·d).

If there is no satisfactory effect after the maximum tolerated dose exceeds 6 weeks, the drug must be stopped.

After symptom control, the dosage was gradually reduced by 0.5~1mg/(kg·d) every 2 weeks until the minimum effective maintenance dose.

Treatment strategies: intermittent short-course therapy, continuous long-range therapy, rescue therapy, alternate therapy, weekend therapy.

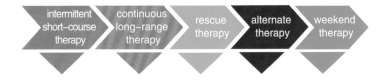

Expected therapeutic effect

Cyclosporine 2.5~5.0mg/(kg·d) for psoriasis for 16 weeks, the response rate of PASI 50, PASI 75 and PASI 90 were 94%, 65% and 29%, respectively.

Common adverse reactions

Hypertension, abnormal renal function, tremor, anorexia, nausea, vomiting, hyperlipemia, hirsutism, acne, etc. Blood routine function, liver function, kidney function, blood lipid, serum potassium ion and magnesium ion should be monitored during medication.

Drug interactions

Alopurinol, statins, macrolide antibiotics, and antifungals can increase the plasma concentration of cyclosporine; antiepileptic drugs, isoniazid, and rifampin can reduce the plasma concentration of cyclosporine; the simultaneous use of cyclosporine and statins carries the risk of rhabdomyolysis.

Contraindications

Renal function impairment, hypertension, malignant tumors, etc.

Ultraviolet Phototherapy

Mechanism of action

Ultraviolet phototherapy utilizes specific wavelengths of ultraviolet (UV) light, including both long wave ultraviolet (UVA) and medium wave ultraviolet (UVB), which have immunomodulatory effects and inhibit inflammatory responses.

Indications

Moderate to severe psoriasis vulgaris.

Therapeutic schedule

Narrow Band UVB (NB UVB)

The dosage is adjusted according to the patient's skin color or the minimum amount of erythema on the skin. Treatment is performed 2~3 times a week, with the dosage gradually increasing according to the treatment response. It can be treated in combination with topical drugs and systemic drugs.

UVA (UVA-1, PUVA)

It can be used as one of the treatment methods, but is currently less commonly used.

308nm excimer light

A highly selective phototherapy used for local treatment of psoriasis.

Expected therapeutic effect

After 4 weeks of NB-UVB treatment, >70% of patients showed significant improvement. A meta-analysis showed that the compliance rate of NB-UVB treatment for PASI 75 was 62%.

Common adverse reactions

Skin dryness, peeling, redness, pigmentation, and in severe cases, pain, blisters, etc.

Contraindications

Absolute contraindications

Congenital diseases with photosensitivity and genetic diseases that may combine or lead to skin cancer.

Relative contraindications

Patients with photosensitive skin diseases, a history of melanoma, organ transplantation receiving immunosuppressive therapy, and those with high risk factors for skin cancer such as arsenic poisoning.

Other suggestions

It is recommended to receive treatment under the guidance of a doctor. If using photosensitive drugs or food, the doctor should be informed.

Topical medication

Classification, name, mechanism of action and clinical application of topical drugs for the treatment of psoriasis vulgaris (Table 3.1).

Table 3.1 Classification, name, mechanism of action and clinical application of topical drugs for psoriasis vulgaris

Classification		Names	Mechanism of action	Therapeutic effects	Method of use	Adverse reactions	Contraindications
Glucocorticoids	super potent	0.02%~ 0.05% clobetasol propionate ointment, etc	Anti–hyperplasia; Anti–inflammation; Immunosuppression	Effective in 1~2 days and significantly improved after 1 week of medication	1~2 times daily; Treatment period < 2 weeks and less than 50g per week	Local reactions: skin atrophy, telangiectasia, hypertrichosis, infection, etc.; Systemic reactions: Hypothalamic–pituitary–adrenal axis inhibition	Allergy to drug ingredients; Skin infections and atrophy
	potent	0.05% halometasone cream, etc					
	Moderately potent	0.1% hydrocortisone butyrate ointment, etc					
	Weakly potent	0.05% desonide cream, etc					
Vitamin D_3 Derivatives		0.005% carpotriol ointment/liniment	Anti–hyperplasia Promote differentiation Immune regulation	The efficacy time is1~ 2 weeks and improves significantly after 4 to 6 weeks of medication	2 times daily; Intermittent treatment period < 1 year; Continued treatment < 20 weeks, less than 100g per week	Local skin irritation; And reversible serum calcium elevation	Allergic to drug ingredients; People with abnormal calcium metabolism
		0.0002% Tacathinol ointment					
Retinoids		0.1%, 0.05% Tazarotene cream/gel	Anti–inflammation Immune regulation	Better efficacy after 12 weeks; or re moval of skin lesions	1 time daily	Local skin irritation; Light sensitivity	Allergic to drug ingredients; Women who are pregnant, planning pregnancy, or lactating
Calcineurin inhibitor		1% Pimecrolimus cream	Anti–inflammation Immune regulation	Efficacy time after 2 weeks, skin lesions basically subsided in more than half of the patients at 8 weeks	2 times daily		
		0.03%, 0.1% tacrolimus ointment					

con.

Classification	Names	Mechanism of action	Therapeutic effects	Method of use	Adverse reactions	Contraindications
Keratinizing agents	3% salicylic acid cream, 10% urea cream, etc	Promoting differentiation	Restore skin barrier, Adjuvant therapy	1 to 2 times daily	Local skin irritation	Allergic to drug ingredients; Salicylic acid above 5% concentration is not used in pregnant and lactating women
Keratolytic agents	5%~10% salicylic acid cream, 20%~40% urea cream, etc	anti-proliferation Exfoliating				
Compound preparations	Calcipotriol betamethasone ointment	Anti-proliferation Promoting differentiation Anti-inflammatory	PASI decreased by 39.2% and 71.3% after 1 week and 4 weeks, respectively	1 time daily, Continued treatment <16 weeks, intermittent treatment < 1 year	Skin irritation, telangiectasia, infection, atrophy, hypercalcemia, adrenal cortex depression	Allergic to drug ingredients; Patients with calcium metabolism disorder; Skin infection and atrophy
	Tazarotene betamethasone cream	Immunosuppression Immune regulation	The effective rate was 65.0% after 4 weeks	1 time daily, Less than 45g per week, and the treatment period was 4–8 weeks	Skin irritation, dryness, desquamation, skin infection, atrophy, telangiectasia, adrenal cortex depression	Allergic to drug ingredients; Women who are pregnant, planning pregnancy or breastfeeding; Skin infection and atrophy
	Compound clobetasol propionate ointment		After 4 weeks, the cure rate was 44.01% and the effective rate was 90.52%	2 times daily. No more than 4 weeks for continued treatment		

Optimal selection and use principles of topical medication

According to the area of skin lesions: BSA<3%, simple topical medication can be considered. BSA≥3%, topical medication combined with systemic therapy, ultraviolet phototherapy, etc.

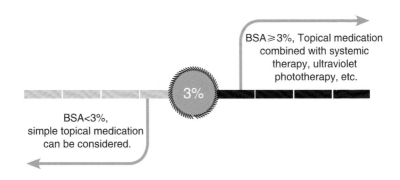

BSA≥3%, Topical medication combined with systemic therapy, ultraviolet phototherapy, etc.

3%

BSA<3%, simple topical medication can be considered.

According to the lesion site

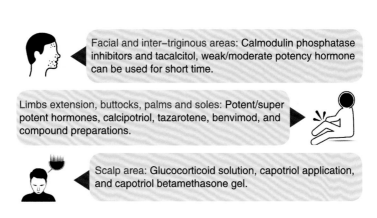

Facial and inter–triginous areas: Calmodulin phosphatase inhibitors and tacalcitol, weak/moderate potency hormone can be used for short time.

Limbs extension, buttocks, palms and soles: Potent/super potent hormones, calcipotriol, tazarotene, benvimod, and compound preparations.

Scalp area: Glucocorticoid solution, capotriol application, and capotriol betamethasone gel.

According to the characteristics of skin lesions

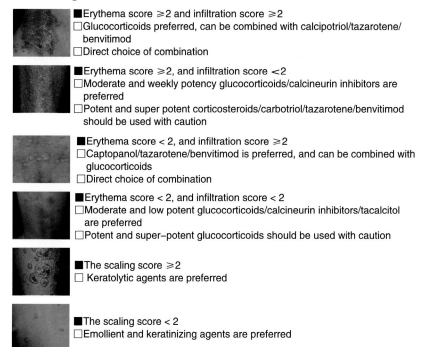

■Erythema score ≥2 and infiltration score ≥2
□Glucocorticoids preferred, can be combined with calcipotriol/tazarotene/benvitimod
□Direct choice of combination

■Erythema score ≥2, and infiltration score <2
□Moderate and weekly potency glucocorticoids/calcineurin inhibitors are preferred
□Potent and super potent corticosteroids/carbotriol/tazarotene/benvitimod should be used with caution

■Erythema score < 2, and infiltration score ≥2
□Captopanol/tazarotene/benvitimod is preferred, and can be combined with glucocorticoids
□Direct choice of combination

■Erythema score < 2, and infiltration score < 2
□Moderate and low potent glucocorticoids/calcineurin inhibitors/tacalcitol are preferred
□Potent and super–potent glucocorticoids should be used with caution

■The scaling score ≥2
□ Keratolytic agents are preferred

■The scaling score < 2
□Emollient and keratinizing agents are preferred

Note: Refer to the attached PASI scores for specific assessment of erythema, infiltration and scaling.

Dose of topical medication

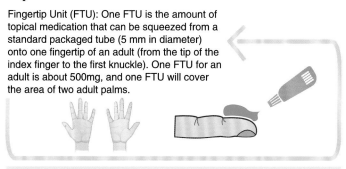

Fingertip Unit (FTU): One FTU is the amount of topical medication that can be squeezed from a standard packaged tube (5 mm in diameter) onto one fingertip of an adult (from the tip of the index finger to the first knuckle). One FTU for an adult is about 500mg, and one FTU will cover the area of two adult palms.

 Special emphasis:

★ potent/super potent hormones should not normally exceed 50g per week and captopanol ointment should not exceed 100g per week.

Frequency of topical medications

Apply topically 1~2 times daily.

Encapsulation therapy

It is suitable for limited, stubborn and hypertrophic skin lesions, which can increase drug penetration and improve curative effect.

Active maintenance therapy

Emollients and keratinizing agents should be continued to use after the skin lesions subsided to prevent recurrence of skin lesions.

Biological Agents and Small Molecular Targeted Drugs

Biological agents

Overview

Currently, the main biological agents used in the treatment of psoriasis include inhibitors of Interleukin (IL) 17, IL–12/23 and IL–23, and inhibitors of Tumour Necrosis Factor alpha (TNF–α). The following provides a brief overview of the mechanisms, indications, pre–treatment screening, efficacy, and safety of these biological agents.

IL–17A inhibitor

IL–17A and its receptor inhibitors approved for the treatment of adult psoriasis vulgaris (Table 3.2)

Table 3.2   Molecular characteristics, indications, usage, efficacy and adverse reactions of IL-17A inhibitors

		(Secukinumab)	(Ixekizumab)	(Brodalumab)
Target		IL-17A	IL-17A	IL17RA
Molecular characteristic		Fully human monoclonal antibody	Humanized monoclonal antibody (98.2% human + 1.8% mouse)	Fully human monoclonal antibody
Indications	Mainland	Patients with moderate to severe plaque psoriasis who meet the criteria for systemic therapy or phototherapy, aged 6 years and above	Adult patients with moderate to severe plaque psoriasis who are candidates for systemic therapy or phototherapy	Not yet on the market
	Taiwan	Patients with moderate to severe plaque psoriasis who meet the criteria for systemic therapy, aged 6 years and above	Patients with moderate to severe plaque psoriasis who meet the criteria for systemic therapy, aged 6 years and above	Adult patients with moderate to severe plaque psoriasis who are candidates for systemic therapy
	Hong Kong and Macao	Patients with moderate to severe plaque psoriasis who need systemic therapy, aged 6 years and above	Adult patients with moderate to severe plaque psoriasis who need systemic therapy	Patients with psoriasis vulgaris who have insufficient response to phototherapy and other existing systemic therapies (except biologics) and patients with a rash area of more than 10%; patients with refractory lesions
Method of administration: subcutaneous injection	Loading Dose	150 mg once a week for 5 consecutive times	First 160mg, then 80mg once every 2 weeks for 7 consecutive times	210mg once a week for 3 consecutive times
	Maintenance	300mg q4w	80mg q4w	210mg q2w

con.

	(Secukinumab)	(Ixekizumab)	(Brodalumab)
Expected efficacy	PASI 90/100 at 12w: 91.7%/39.7% ASI 90/100 at 52 w: 91.1%/68.8% ASI 90/100 at 5 year: 74.5%/47.6%	PASI 90/100 at 12w: 82.4%/33% ASI90/100 at 52W: 84%/64% ASI90/100 at 5 Year: 67.1%/46.2%	PASI 90/100 at 12w: 77.8%/63.3% ASI 90/100 at 52w: 81.8%/72.7.% ASI 90/100 at 2.3 year: 86%/74%
Common adverse reactions	Upper respiratory tract infection such as rhinitis, herpes simplex, fungal infection	Injection site reaction, upper respiratory tract infection such as sore throat, fungal infection, and herpes simplex	Symptoms of influenza such as throat pain, injection site reactions, fungal infections
Contraindications	Allergic to drug ingredients, severe active infections (such as active tuberculosis), inflammatory bowel disease, etc		

IL–12/23 Inhibitors and IL–23 Inhibitors

IL–12/23 inhibitors and IL–23 inhibitors for psoriasis (Table 3.3).

Table 3.3   Molecular characteristics, indications, usage, efficacy and adverse effects of IL–12/23 and IL–23 inhibitors

		Ustekinumab	Guselkumab	Risankizumab
Target of Action		P40 subunit of IL–12/23	P19 subunit of IL–23	P19 subunit of IL–23
Molecular Characteristics		Fully Human		
Indication	Mainland	Adult patients with moderate to severe plaque psoriasis who are candidates for photo-therapy or systemic therapy	Adult patients with moderate to severe psoriasis vulgaris	Moderate to severe psoriasis vulgaris
	Taiwan			
	Hong Kong Macau	Patients aged 6 years old and above with moderate to severe plaque psoriasis	Adult Patients with Moderate to severe plaque psoriasis suitable for systemic therapy	

con.

		Ustekinumab	Guselkumab	Risankizumab
Method of administration: Subcutaneous injection	Induction Period	Week 0 and Week 4, weight ≤ 100kg, 45 mg each time Weight > 100kg, 90 mg each time	100mg each at Week 0 and Week 4	150mg at Week 0 and Week 4
	Maintenance Period	Once every 12 weeks, weight ≤ 100kg, 45mg; weight > 100kg, 90mg	Every 8 weeks 100 mg each time	Every 12 weeks 150mg each time
Expected Efficacy		Week 12–16: PASI 90/100 42%/13% and 37%/11% for 45mg and 90mg groups, respectively Week 48–52: PASI 90 58% and 71% in the 45mg and 90mg groups, respectively 5 years: PASI 90 60%	Week 16: PASI 90/ 100 73%, 37% Week 48: PASI 90/ 100 76.3%, 47.4% 5 years: PASI 90 82%.	Week 16: PASI 90/ 100 75.3%, 35.9% Week 52: PASI 90/ 100 82%, 56% Week 172: PASI 90/ 100 85.5% and 54.4%, respectively
Common Adverse Reactions		Upper respiratory tract infection, headache, etc.	Upper respiratory tract infection, headache, etc.	Upper respiratory tract infection, headache, fungal infection, listless, etc.
Contraindications		Allergy to any component of the drug, serious active infection, etc.		

TNF–α inhibitors

TNF–α inhibitors which have been approved for the treatment of adult patients with psoriasis vulgaris (Table 3.4).

Table 3.4   Molecular characteristics, indications, usage, efficacy, and adverse reactions of TNF–α inhibitors

	Adalimumab	Etanercept	Infliximab
Targets	TNF–α	TNF–α	TNF–α
Molecular characteristics	Recombinant whole human monoclonal antibody	Humanized TNF–α receptor antibody fusion protein	Human–mouse chimeric monoclonal antibody

con.

		Adalimumab	Etanercept	Infliximab
Indication	Chinese Mainland	Adult patients with moderate to severe plaque psoriasis, who require systematic treatment. Severe plaque psoriasis in children over 4 years old	Adult patients with moderate to severe plaque psoriasis	Adult patients with moderate to severe plaque psoriasis, who require systematic treatment. Meanwhile, traditional systemic drugs or phototherapy are ineffective or intolerant
	Taiwan	Adult patients with moderate to severe psoriasis who are ineffective, contraindicated, or intolerable to other systemic treatments or phototherapy		—
	Hong Kong/ Macao	Adult patients with moderate to severe plaque psoriasis		
Medication methods	Induction period	Subcutaneous injection, initial dose 80mg, 40mg in the second week	Subcutaneous injection, 25mg per time, twice a week;	Intravenousinfusion,5mg/kg administered at weeks 0, 2, and 6
	Holding phase	Subcutaneous injection, 40mg every 2 weeks	or 50mg per time, once a week	Intravenous infusion, 5mg/kg administered every 8 weeks
Expected Efficacy		12 weeks: PASI 75 ranges from 58.7% to 77.8%, and PASI90 ranges from 30.43% 52 weeks: PASI 75/90 are 73.3% and 60.4%, respectively 160 weeks: PASI 75/90 are 76% and 50% respectively	12 weeks: PASI 75/ 90 are 40.98% and 21% respectively 24 weeks: PASI 75 is 66.3% 3 years: PASI 75 is 88.2%	12 weeks: PASI 75/90 are 40.98% and 21% respectively 24 weeks: PASI 75 is 66.3% 3 years: PASI 75 is 88.2%
Common adverse reactions		Upper respiratory tract infection, injection site reaction, lupus like syndrome, etc	Upper respiratory tract infection, injection site reaction, headache, etc	Upper respiratory tract infections, infusion reactions, serum disease like reactions, congestive heart failure, etc

con.

	Adalimumab	Etanercept	Infliximab
Contraindication	Individuals who are allergic to drug; Active pulmonary tuberculosis; moderate to severe congestive heart failure		

Screening and monitoring

Pre-medication examination of biological agents and monitoring indicators during medication (Table 3.5)

Table 3.5 Pre-medication examination and monitoring indicators of biological agents

Examination items	Pre-medication	During medication
Routine analysis of blood and urine; liver function	√	The 4th week, 12th week, and then test every 3 months
Kidney function	√	No special requirements
Hepatitis B and Hepatitis C serological testing	√	Positive individuals: Test every 3~6 months
HIV serological testing	Depending on the patient's condition	No special requirements
antinuclear antibody (ANA)	TNF- α inhibitor	TNF- α Inhibitors: test every 6 months
Tuberculosis screening（PPD or T-spot or QuantiFERON-TB Gold）	√	TNF- α Inhibitors: test every 6 months; other biological agents: test every 12 months
Chest X-ray or CT examination	√	TNF- α Inhibitors: test every 6 months; other biological agents: test every 12 months
Cancer screening	Depending on the patient's condition	No special requirements

HIV, human immunodeficiency virus; T-SPOT, T cell spot detection; TNF-α, Tumor necrosis factor-α;PPD, Pure protein derivative test of tuberculin.

Usage of Biologics for Special Populations （Table 3.6）

Table 3.6　Recommendations for the use of biologics in special populations

Special populations	Medication recommendations
Pregnancy and lactation	Weigh the pros and cons and use carefully if necessary
Tuberculosis patients	TNF–α inhibitors are contraindicated in active tuberculosis; Patients with inactive tuberculosis and latent infection of tuberculosis will be consulted by the infectious disease department to decide whether to give preventive anti tuberculosis treatment
HBV–infected patients	Quantification of HBV–DNA in blood and monitoring of liver function are needed when necessary; Once HBV reactivation is detected, it should be treated as HBV active infection and treated by the infectious disease department
Patients with malignancy	Prohibited for active tumors; It can be applied to tumor patients who have been stable for ⩾ 5 years after treatment; Close monitoring is required, and the pros and cons should be considered before deciding whether to administer the medication
Surgical patients	Medium–to–high risk surgery, discontinue biologics for 3~5 half–lives before undergoing elective surgery; The use of biologics in low–risk surgical patients is not affected
Vaccine Inoculation	Avoid receiving live vaccines during adult medication; For those who use biologics after 16 weeks of gestation, their delivered infants should avoid receiving live vaccines within 6 months after birth
Patients with inflammatory bowel disease	Not suitable for choosing IL–17A inhibitors
Other special populations	Consult the doctor

Small–molecule Targeted Drugs

Apremilast

Mechanism of action

Apremilast specifically inhibits phosphodiesterase 4 (PDE4), blocking the degradation of cyclic adenosine monophosphate (cAMP), which in turn inhibits the synthesis and release of pro-inflammatory factors.

Indications

As the world's first small-molecule oral drug approved to target PDE4 for the treatment of psoriasis, it is also approved in Chinese mainland for the treatment of adult patients with moderate-to-severe plaque psoriasis who are candidates for photo-therapy or systemic therapy.

Therapeutic schedule

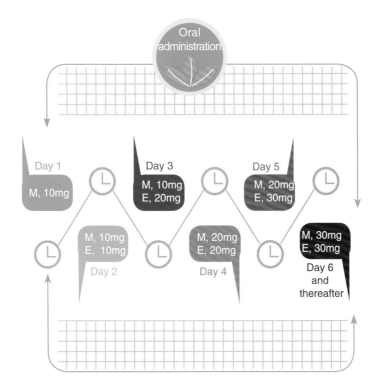

Expected therapeutic effect

The PASI75 response rates were 33.1%, 35%, and 61% at 16, 32, and 52 weeks of treatment, respectively.

Common adverse reactions

Diarrhea, nausea, and vomiting, etc., mostly mild to moderate, often occurred in the first 2 weeks of treatment and mostly resolved within 1 month. In case of unexplained weight loss, assessment shall be performed, and discontinuation of the product shall be considered if necessary.

Drug interactions

It is not recommended to be used in combination with drugs including rifampicin, phenobarbital, carbamazepine, and phenytoin sodium.

Contraindications

It is contraindicated in case of hypersensitivity to apremilast or any of the excipients in the formulation. It is essential to weigh the risks and benefits for patients with a history of depression and/or suicidal ideation or behavior.

Deucravacitinib

Mechanism of action

Deucravacitinib is an oral selective allosteric inhibitor of tyrosine Tyrosine-protein kinase 2 (TYK2), treating psoriasis by precisely blocking the immune inflammation mediated by IL-23, IL-12 and Type I interferons.

Indications

It is indicated for the treatment of moderate-to-severe plaque psoriasis in adults who are candidates for systemic therapy or phototherapy.

Therapeutic schedule

Oral medication of one tablet (6mg) daily.

Expected therapeutic effect

PASI75 response rate at 16 weeks of treatment was 68.8%, and ss-PGA 0/1 response rate was 64%. PASI75 and PASI90 response rates at 52 weeks of treatment were 71.0% and 45.5%, respectively, with durable response and stable efficacy without attenuation.

Common adverse reactions

Nasopharyngitis, upper respiratory tract infection.

Benverimod cream

Mechanism of action

Benvilimod targets aromatic hydrocarbon receptors, effectively regulates the expression of related immune cells and inflammatory factors, acts directly on keratinocytes, and inhibits angiogenesis and telangiectasia.

Indications

Adult mild to moderate stable psoriasis vulgaris suitable for topical treatment.

Therapeutic schedule

Use externally once in the morning and once in the evening. It is not recommended to rub the head, face, groin, anus, etc. The maximum daily dose is less than 6g, and the treatment area is less than 10% of the body surface area. Avoid UV exposure to the application area.

Expected therapeutic effect

At 12 weeks of treatment, the PASI 75 compliance rate was 50.4%.

Common adverse reactions

Redness, itching, contact dermatitis, folliculitis, pigmentation abnormalities, etc. at the site of application are mostly transient and mild to moderate, and can mostly improve on their own.

Drug interactions

It's not clear yet.

Contraindications

Those who are allergic to any of the ingredients in this product are prohibited; pregnant, planning pregnancy, and breastfeeding women are prohibited; erythrodermic psoriasis, generalized pustular psoriasis, etc. are prohibited.

Traditional Chinese Medicine and Chinese Materia Medica

Etiology and pathogenesis

Psoriasis, known as 'White Crust' in Traditional Chinese Medicine (TCM), is a cutaneous disease caused by constitutional heat, or external infection of pathogens, or emotions injury, or irregular diets, leading to stagnation of qi movement. Chronic or recurrent course of psoriasis may deplete yin–blood, then foster dryness and cause wind. Yin–blood deficiencies further induce meridian obstruction, qi and blood stagnation, result in skin malnutrition.

Types of syndromes

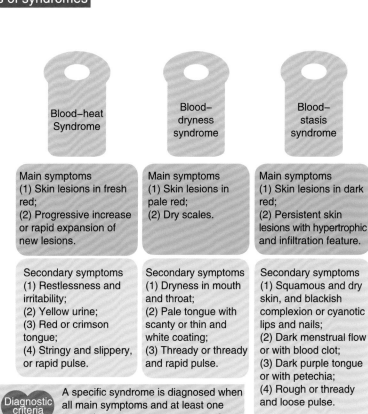

Blood–heat Syndrome

Main symptoms
(1) Skin lesions in fresh red;
(2) Progressive increase or rapid expansion of new lesions.

Secondary symptoms
(1) Restlessness and irritability;
(2) Yellow urine;
(3) Red or crimson tongue;
(4) Stringy and slippery, or rapid pulse.

Blood– dryness syndrome

Main symptoms
(1) Skin lesions in pale red;
(2) Dry scales.

Secondary symptoms
(1) Dryness in mouth and throat;
(2) Pale tongue with scanty or thin and white coating;
(3) Thready or thready and rapid pulse.

Blood– stasis syndrome

Main symptoms
(1) Skin lesions in dark red;
(2) Persistent skin lesions with hypertrophic and infiltration feature.

Secondary symptoms
(1) Squamous and dry skin, and blackish complexion or cyanotic lips and nails;
(2) Dark menstrual flow or with blood clot;
(3) Dark purple tongue or with petechia;
(4) Rough or thready and loose pulse.

Diagnostic criteria A specific syndrome is diagnosed when all main symptoms and at least one secondary symptom are presented.

Syndrome differentiation and treatment principles

Distinct syndrome types necessitate disparate treatment principles, methods, and prescriptions.

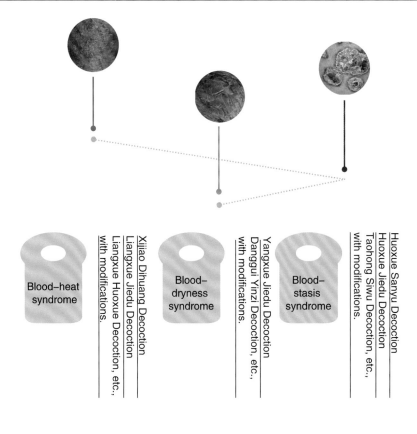

Blood–heat syndrome

Xijiao Dihuang Decoction
Liangxue Jiedu Decoction
Liangxue Huoxue Decoction, etc.,
with modifications.

Blood–dryness syndrome

Yangxue Jiedu Decoction
Danggui Yinzi Decoction, etc.,
with modifications.

Blood–stasis syndrome

Huoxue Sanyu Decoction
Huoxue Jiedu Decoction
Taohong Siwu Decoction, etc.,
with modifications.

Oral Chinese patent medicines

Blood–heat syndrome

Compound Qingdai (Capsule, Pill, Tablet),
Xiaoyin (Granule, Capsule, Tablet),
Yinxie Capsule, Keyin Pill,
Baixuan Xiatare Tablet, etc.

Blood–dryness syndrome

Xiaoyin (Capsule, Pill, Tablet),
Zidan Yinxie Capsule,
Runzao Zhiyang Capsule, etc.

Blood–stasis syndrome

Yujin Yinxie Tablet,
Yinxie Capsule, etc.

Precautions

Contraindicated in individuals with known allergies to these medicines.

Caution advised in children, the elderly, pregnant, or lactating women.

Pay attention to the treatment course of bitter and cold medicine to prevent adverse effects on the spleen and stomach.

During medication, avoidance of smoking, alcohol, spicy and greasy foods, and irritating or allergenic substances.

Adverse reactions

diarrhea, abdominal pain, nausea, vomiting, and sporadic rash and pruritus.

TCM External Treatment and non–pharmacological therapy

Tailored TCM external treatments, such as medicated bathing, medicated compressing, fumigation, inunction and medicated wrapping, are applied based on syndrome differentiation. Non–pharmacological therapies cover retained cupping, flash cupping, moving cupping, blood–letting cupping, acupuncture, thread embedding at acupoints, fire needle, moxibustion, three–edged needle, and ear acupuncture. TCM therapeutic modalities, with their versatility and absence of toxic side effects, enhance efficacy and impede disease recurrence.

TCM regulation

Adherence to a rational diet, avoiding undue dietary restrictions, and controlled dieting for overweight or obese individuals. Abstain from smoking and moderating alcohol intake. Maintain regular sleep patterns and ensure emotional well–being. Obey the principle of "nourishing yang in spring and summer, nourishing yin in autumn and winter" during the remission period. Practice exercises such as Ba Duan Jin and Five Animals Exercise for bodily relaxation. In the early recovery stage, appropriate medication for nourishing blood, nourishing yin, and regulating the spleen and stomach should be used to consolidate the therapeutic effect. Avoiding six pathogenic factors, as well as conditioning body, which promotes rehabilitations after skin lesions regression.

The Mechanism of Drug Action

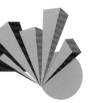

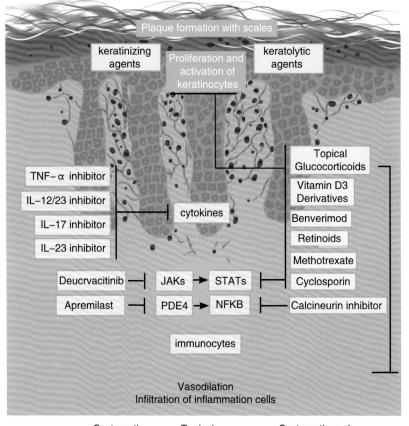

The mechanism of drug action

Chapter 4

Testing the Patient´s Understanding of
the Basic Decision−making Process

How serious do you think your psoriasis is? (single choice)

□Mild   □Moderate   □Severe

Have you decided which treatment to choose? (Optional)

( ) Topical medicine

( ) Traditional systemic medication:

 □Methotrexate   □Cyclosporin   □Acitretin

( ) Traditional Chinese medicine

( ) Phototherapy

( ) Biological agents: □Sikuchizumab   □Ikizumab

 □Gusechizumab   □Adalimumab

 □Infliximab   □Risankizumab

 □Others

( ) Small molecule drugs: □Apremilast   □Deuteroclexitinib

 □Benvitimod

( ) I'd like to think about it some more

If your condition becomes worse during treatment, which of the following treatment options will you choose? (single choice)

□increase the dosage by oneself

□learn the treatment experience from the fellow patients

□go to the hospital and adjust the treatment plan under the guidance of the doctor

What are the important precautions for the application of biologics? (multiple choices)

□strict screening before medication

□drug safety monitoring should be conducted regularly during medication

□the adjustment of dosage and interval should be carried out under the guidance of the doctor

□self drug withdrawal if the rashes dissipate

Appendix A

Body Surface Area (BSA) scoring

The flexion area of a patient's single palm and finger was defined as 1% of the body surface area, and the total number of palm areas of the patient's total body lesions was assessed, which was recorded as BSA. Please refer to the following ratios when evaluating:

Head and neck =10% body surface area (10 palms)

Upper limbs =20% body surface area (20 palms)

Trunk (including armpits and groin) = 30% body surface area (30 palms)

Lower limbs (including buttocks) = 40% body surface area (40 palms)

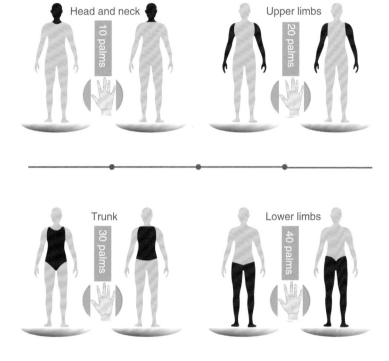

Appendix B

Psoriasis Area and Severity Index (PASI) Scoring

The PASI scoring criteria include the area score and the severity score. It is an important indicator to evaluate the severity of psoriasis, and it is also an indicator to quantify the severity of psoriasis, reflecting the condition of psoriasis with a specific number, with a score between 0 and 72. The higher the score, the wider the range of lesions and the serious lesions (figue B.1).

Severity of psoriasis lesions				
0=no lesion，1=mild，2=moderate，3=severe，4=very severe				
	head	trunk	upper limbs	lower limbs
red spot	0~4	0~4	0~4	0~4
thickness	0~4	0~4	0~4	0~4
scale	0~4	0~4	0~4	0~4
total ①	Sum of the above scores	Sum of the above scores	Sum of the above scores	Sum of the above scores
Area of psoriasis lesions				
0=no lesion；1<10%; 2=10~29%; 3=30~49%;4=50~69%; 5=70~89%; 6=90~100%				
Involved area score ②	0~6	0~6	0~6	0~6
①×②	①×②	①×②	①×②	①×②
Body part coefficient	0.1	0.3	0.2	0.4
①×②×③	A	B	C	D
PASI=A+B+C+D (0~72)				

figue B.1 PASI scoring

Appendix C

Dermatology Life Quality Index (DLQI) Questionnaire

The DLQI score is a quality of life score for patients with psoriasis, mainly through questionnaires to understand the impact of psoriasis on patients' daily life.

DLQI questionnaire has 10 questions, each question has 4 different answers, respectively, no, slight, serious, extremely serious, corresponding score values are 0, 1, 2, 3 points, and finally add the 10 score values to get the total DLQI score value (degree rating: 0~1, no impact; 2~5 points, mild; 6 to 10 points, moderate; > 10 points, severe.

DLQI questionnaire

The following questions are to find out how much of an impact your skin problem has had on your life in the past week.

1. Has your skin been itchy, tender, sore, or tingling in the last week?	☐ quite a lot ☐ a lot of ☐a little ☐not at all
2. In the last week, have you felt embarrassed or low self-esteem due to your skin problem?	☐quite a lot ☐ a lot of ☐a little ☐not at all
3. In the last week, how did your skin problem affect your shopping, housework, and yard work?	☐quite a lot ☐ a lot of ☐a little ☐not at all
4. How has your skin problem affected your clothing in the last week?	☐quite a lot ☐ a lot of ☐a little ☐not at all
5. In the last week, how much has the skin problem affected your social or leisure life?	☐quite a lot ☐ a lot of ☐a little ☐not at all
6. How much your skin problem has hindered your exercise in the last week?	☐quite a lot ☐ a lot of ☐a little ☐not at all
7. Have you had skin problems that prevented you from going to work or studying in the last week?	☐quite a lot ☐ a lot of ☐a little ☐not at all
8. Has your skin condition prevented you from interacting with a loved one, close friend, or relatives in the last week?	☐quite a lot ☐ a lot of ☐a little ☐not at all
9. How your skin problem has affected your sex life in the last week?	☐quite a lot ☐ a lot of ☐a little ☐not at all
10. How much trouble have it caused you in the last week by treating your skin problems, such as making a mess around the house or taking up a lot of your time?	☐quite a lot ☐ a lot of ☐a little ☐not at all

Appendix D

Investigator´s Global Assessment (IGA)

IGA is one of the most commonly used assessment indicators in clinical studies of dermatology to assess the severity of a patient's condition and the effect of treatment. This evaluation method can help doctors and researchers better assess the overall condition and outcome of patients, and provide quantitative evaluation results (Table D.1) .

Table D.1　IGA

score	Short description	Detailed description
0	recession	no symptoms of psoriasis; post-inflammatory pigmentation may be present
1	almost recession	normal to pink lesions; no thickening; no or very slight focal scale
2	mild	pink to reddish skin lesions; mild thickening, mild scaling can be detected
3	moderate	dark bright red, clearly discernible erythema, clearly discernible to moderate thickening, medium scale
4	severe	Bright to deep dark red, heavily thickened with hard edges, almost all or all of the lesions covered with heavy/coarse scales

Appendix E

Index of Matrix

English Full Name	English Abbreviation
Acitretin	
Adalimumab	
body surface area	BSA
Brodalumab	
Cyclosporin	
dermatology life quality index	DLQI
Deucravacitinib	
Etanercept	
fingertip unit	FTU
Guselkumab	
infliximab	
interleukin	IL
investigator's global assessment	IGA
Ixekizumab	
Methotrexate	MTX
narrow band UVB	NB-UVB
phosphodiesterase	PDE4
psoriasis area severity index	PASI
Risankizumab	
Secukinumab	
scalp-specific physician's global assessment	ss-PGA
tumour necrosis factor-α	TNF-α
ultraviolet	UV
Ustekinumab	

References

1.CHEN XIAOLAN, ZHENG LIYING, ZHANG HAO,et al. Investigation of disease burden and quality of life in patients with psoriasis: a web-based questionnaire survey[J]. Chinese Journal of Dermatology, 2019, 52(11):791-795.

2.PSORIASIS COMMITTEE OF CHINESE SOCIETY OF DERMATOLOGY. Chinese guideline for the diagnosis and treatment of psoriasis (2023 edition) [J]. Chinese Journal of Dermatology, 2023, 56(7):573-625.

3.PSORIASIS GROUP OF CHINESE SOCIETY OF DERMATOLOGY. Expert guidance on the treatment of psoriasis with Benvitimod cream[J]. Chinese Journal of Dermatology, 2021, 35(6): 707-711.

4.ZHAO BINGNAN, ZHANG ZHILI. Concise Dermatology in Traditional Chinese Medicine [M]. Beijing: China Press of Traditional Chinese Medicine, 2014: 190.

5.DERMATOLOGY BRANCH OF CHINA ASSOCIATION OF CHINESE MEDICINE. Expert Consensus on the Psoriasis Treatment of TCM (2017 Edition) [J]. Chinese Journal of Dermatovenereology of Integrated Traditional and Western Medicine, 2018, 17(3): 273-277.

6.CHEN ZHAOXIA, LI PING, ZHANG GUANGZHONG, et al. Moxibustion Treatment on Plaque Psoriasis with Blood Stasis Syndrome: A Randomized Controlled Trail[J]. Chinese Acupuncture, 2021, 41(7): 762-766.

7.KOMINE M, KIM H, YI J, et al. A discrete choice experiment on oral and injection treatment preferences among moderate-to-severe psoriasis patients in Japan[J]. J Dermatol,2023,50(6): 766-777.

8.LEE JH, YOUN JI, KIM TY, et al. A multicenter, randomized, open-label pilot trial assessing the efficacy and safety of etanercept 50 mg twice weekly followed by etanercept 25 mg twice weekly, the combination of etanercept 25 mg twice weekly and acitretin, and acitretin alone in patients with moderate to severe psoriasis[J]. BMC Dermatol,2016,16 (1):11.

9.DOGRA S, JAIN A, KANWAR AJ. Efficacy and safety of acitretin in three fixed doses of 25, 35 and 50 mg in adult patients with severe plaque type psoriasis: a randomized, double blind, parallel group, dose ranging study[J]. J Eur Acad Dermatol Venereol,2013,27:e305-311.

10.YU C, FAN X, LI Z, et al. Efficacy and safety of total glucosides of paeony combined with acitretin in the treatment of moderate-to-severe plaque psoriasis: a double-blind, randomised, placebo-controlled trial[J]. Eur J Dermatol,2017,27:150-154.

11.WARREN RB, MROWIETZ U, VON KIEDROWSKI R, et al. An intensified dosing schedule of subcutaneous methotrexate in patients with moderate to severe plaque-type psoriasis (METOP): a 52 week, multicentre, randomised, double-blind, placebo-controlled, phase 3 trial[J]. Lancet,2017,389(10068):528-537.

12.CHEN TJ, CHUNG WH, CHEN CB, et al. Methotrexate-induced epidermal necrosis: A case series of 24 patients[J]. J Am Acad Dermatol,2017,77(2):247-255.

13.RICHARDS HL, FORTUNE DG, O'SULLIVAN TM, et al. Patients with psoriasis and their compliance with medication[J]. J Am Acad Dermatol,1999,41(4):581-583.

14.HO VC, GRIFFITHS CE, BERTH-JONES J, et al. Intermittent short courses of cyclosporine microemulsion for the long-term management of psoriasis: a 2-year cohort study[J]. J Am Acad Dermatol,2001, 44 (4): 643-651.

15.ELMETS CA, LIM HW, STOFF B, et al. Joint American Academy of Dermatology-National Psoriasis Foundation guidelines of care for the management and treatment of psoriasis with phototherapy[J]. J Am Acad Dermatol,2019,81(3):775-804.

16.GOULDEN V, LING TC, BABAKINEJAD P, et al. British Association of Dermatologistsapy. J Am Acad Dermatol. 2019;81(3):775-8ation of Dermatologists and British Photodermatology Group guidelines for narrowband ultraviolet B phototherapy 2022[J]. Br J Dermatol, 2022,187(3):295-308.

17.DANIEL BS, ORCHARD D. Ocular side-effects of topical corticosteroids: what a dermatologist needs to know[J]. Australas J Dermatol,2015,56(3): 164-169.

18.SMITH SH, JAYAWICKREME C, RICKARD DJ, et al. Tapinarof Is a Natural AhR Agonist that Resolves Skin Inflammation in Mice and Humans[J]. J Invest Dermatol,2017,137(10): 2110-2119.

19.ZHOU J, YUAN Y, LIU Y, et al. Effectiveness and safety of secukinumab in Chinese patients with moderate to severe plaque psoriasis in real-world practice[J]. Exp Dermatol, 2023. doi:10.1111/exd.14890.

20.LI XIA, ZHENG JIE, PAN WEI-LI, et al. Efficacy and Safety of Ixekizumab in Chinese Patients with Moderate-to-Severe Plaque Psoriasis: 60-Week Results From a Phase 3 Study [J]. International journal of Dermatology and Venereology,2022,5(4):181-190.

21.BLAUVELT A, LEBWOHL MG, MABUCHI T, et al. Long-term efficacy and safety of ixekizumab: A 5-year analysis of the UNCOVER-3 randomized controlled trial[J]. J Am Acad Dermatol,2021,85(2):360-368.

22.GALLUZZO M, CALDAROLA G, SIMONE CD, et al. Use of brodalumab for the treatment of chronic plaque psoriasis: a one-year real-life study in the Lazio region, Italy[J]. Expert

Opin Biol Ther,2021,21(9):1299-1310.

23.LEONARDI CL, KIMBALL AB, PAPP KA, et al. Efficacy and safety of ustekinumab, a human interleukin-12/23 monoclonal antibody, in patients with psoriasis: 76-week results from a randomised, double-blind, placebo-controlled trial (PHOENIX 1) [J]. Lancet,2008, 371(9625):1665-1674.

24.PAPP KA, GRIFFITHS CE, GORDON K, et al. Long-term safety of ustekinumab in patients with moderate-to-severe psoriasis: final results from 5 years of follow-up[J]. Br J Dermatol,2013,168(4):844-854.

25.BLAUVELT A, PAPP KA, GRIFFITHS CEM, et al. Efficacy and safety of guselkumab, an anti-interleukin-23 monoclonal antibody, compared with adalimumab for the continuous treatment of patients with moderate to severe psoriasis: Results from the phase III, double-blinded, placebo- and active comparator-controlled VOYAGE 1 trial[J]. J Am Acad Dermatol,2017,76(3):405-417.

26.GORDON KB, STROBER B, LEBWOHL M, et al. Efficacy and safety of risankizumab in moderate-to-severe plaque psoriasis (UltIMMa-1 and UltIMMa-2): results from two double-blind, randomised, placebo-controlled and ustekinumab-controlled phase 3 trials [J]. Lancet,2018,392(10148):650-661.

27.LI GJ, GU YX, ZOU Q, et al. Efficacy, Safety, and Pharmacoeconomic Analysis of Adalimumab and Secukinumab for Moderate-to-Severe Plaque Psoriasis: A Single-Center, Real-World Study[J].Dermatol Ther,2022,12(9):2105-2115.

28.XIE F, WANG R, ZHAO ZG, et al. Safety and efficacy of etanercept monotherapy for moderate-to-severe plaque psoriasis: A prospective 12-week follow-up study[J]. Journal of Huazhong University of Science and Technology,2017,37(6):943-947.

29.PAUL C, CATHER J, GOODERHAM M, et al. Efficacy and safety of apremilast, an oral phosphodiesterase 4 inhibitor, in patients with moderate-to-severe plaque psoriasis over 52 weeks: a phase III, randomized controlled trial(ESTEEM 2)[J]. Br J Dermatol,2015,173(6): 1387-1399.

30.ARMSTRONG AW, GOODERHAM M, WARREN RB, et al. Deucravacitinib versus placebo and apremilast in moderate to severe plaque psoriasis: efficacy and safety results from the 52-week, randomized, double-blinded, placebo-controlled phase 3 POETYK PSO-1 trial[J]. J Am Acad Dermatol,2023,88(1):29-39.

31.CAI L, CHEN GH, LU QJ, et al. A double-blind, randomized, placebo- and positive-controlled phase III trial of 1% benvitimod cream in mild-to-moderate plaque psoriasis[J]. Chin Med J,2020,133(24):2905-2909.

Acknowledgments

This consensus is the crystallization of the collective wisdom of dermatologists across the Taiwan Strait and in Hong Kong and Macao regions. It has received attention and support from all members of the Psoriasis Professional Committee of the Cross-Strait Medical Health Exchange Association. Academician Liao Wanqing is happy to preface the consensus, which fully reflect the strong support and high recognition of the consensus by predecessors in the academic community.

Mr. Ke Yimou, Chairman of Taiwan Association of Psoriasis, Mr. Li Qingkun, President of Hong Kong Psoriasis Patients Association, Mr. Shi Xingxiang, Initiator of Mainland Mutual Assistance of Psoriasis Patient Website, Ms. Wang Yaxin, Secretary-General of Taiwan Association of Psoriasis, and other representatives of psoriasis patients across the Strait and from Hong Kong and Macao also put forward valuable opinions and suggestions on the content of the consensus, so that the purpose of doctor-patient joint decision-making is well achieved.

The visually informative presentation of this consensus owes much to the diligent efforts of Wang Lihua.

President Wang Liji and other leaders of the Cross-Strait Medical Health Exchange Association have provided strong support and guidance for the successful publication of this consensus.

Dr. Gao Yunlu from Shanghai Skin Disease Hospital, Dr. Guo Liping from the Department of Dermatology, Erdos Central Hospital, and Dr. Wang Xiaoyu from the Department of Dermatology, Peking University Third Hospital have provided strong support and assistance in the writing and translation of this consensus.

Here, we would like to express our most sincere gratitude to all the leaders, colleagues, and friends who have provided assistance to the creation of this consensus!